The integration of behavioural and cognitive approaches to psychotherapy has much to offer in the treatment of a wide range of disabling conditions in psychiatry. In this book the authors, both experienced clinicians and teachers, provide what they describe as a 'tool-kit' for the management of patients using behavioural and cognitive psychotherapy.

Based firmly on the work of the pioneers of behavioural and cognitive approaches, the authors illustrate the application of these principles through a vivid and instructive series of case histories. They show how, properly applied, behavioural and cognitive psychotherapy can contribute to the treatment and rehabilitation of even severely incapacitated patients. The cases discussed range from obsessive compulsive disorders and anxiety states through to chronically disabled patients with schizophrenia or depression. Chapters are also devoted to the use of these techniques in marital therapy, sex therapy, social skills training and the treatment of psychosomatic disorders. A comprehensive glossary of terms used in behavioural and cognitive therapy is provided for newcomers to this field.

Always the emphasis is on practical work with patients for the alleviation of maladaptive or unwanted behaviour and thoughts, and the authors also give guidance on some of the pitfalls to be avoided and on the concomitant use of medication. This book will, therefore, be of value to all mental health professionals training in the use of behavioural and cognitive psychotherapy.

The Practice of Behavioural and Cognitive Psychotherapy

The Practice of Behavioural and Cognitive Psychotherapy

RICHARD S. STERN MD, FRC Psych.

Consultant Psychiatrist, St George's Hospital, London and St Helier Hospital, Surrey
Honorary Senior Lecturer in Psychiatry, St George's Hospital Medical School, London

LYNNE M. DRUMMOND MRCP, MRC Psych.

Consultant Psychiatrist and Senior Lecturer in Behavioural Psychotherapy,
St George's Hospital Medical School, London

Illustrations by
MANDY ASSIN, MB, BS, MRC Psych.

Registrar in Psychiatry, St George's Hospital , London

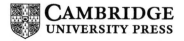
CAMBRIDGE
UNIVERSITY PRESS

Published by the Press Syndicate of the University of Cambridge
The Pitt Building, Trumpington Street, Cambridge CB2 1RP
40 West 20th Street, New York, NY 10011–4211, USA
10 Stamford Road, Oakleigh, Melbourne 3166, Australia

First published 1991
Reprinted 1995

Printed in Great Britain by Bell & Bain Ltd, Glasgow

British Library cataloguing in publication data

Stern, Richard
The practice of behavioural and cognitive psychotherapy.
1. Psychotherapy
I. Title   II. Drummond, Lynne M.
616.8914

Library of Congress cataloguing in publication data

Stern, Richard
The practice of behavioural and cognitive psychotherapy / Richard Stern,
Lynne M. Drummond; illustrations by Mandy Assin.
    p.   cm.
Includes bibliographical references.
Includes index
ISBN 0 521 38742 6 (pb)
1. Cognitive therapy.   2. Behavior therapy.   I. Drummond, Lynne M.   II. Title.
[DNLM: 1. Behavior Therapy – methods.   2. Cognitive Therapy – methods.
WM 425 S839P]
RC489.C63S74   1991
616.89'142—dc20   91-8015   CIP

ISBN 0 521 38742 6 paperback

PN

Contents

Foreword by Professor Isaac Marks

Behavioural treatment has come of age. It is an efficient approach to help many sufferers overcome a wide range of problems and resume living normal lives. There are still too few easy guides to behavioural treatment for would-be therapists, so this new book is very welcome. Practitioners of behavioural treatment need such how-to-do-it guidance more than learned theoretical disquisitions. In this easy-to-read volume they will find a wide variety of case histories of therapy in sufficiently rich detail to apply similar principles to their own cases. It contains many clinical examples of sensitive treatment applications which will encourage practitioners to hone their own skills according to the needs of their particular patients.

The behavioural field is developing rapidly. One important advance concerns self-help for anxiety disorders. Self-exposure is now known to be so successful that, as this book notes, in the great majority of people with anxiety disorders clinician-accompanied exposure is unnecessary. The therapist's main task is to act as coach encouraging the patient to work out and complete appropriate exposure targets and monitoring progress towards their achievement. Stern and Drummond give clear guidance on this topic.

Also mentioned here is the recent NIMH multicentre controlled study of the treatment of depression. In that study interpersonal therapy was at least as effective as cognitive therapy. The cognitive part of cognitive therapy may be redundant, the core element to the various successful brief psychotherapies for depression being task-oriented problem-solving.

Other new knowledge relates to medication with exposure in some sufferers with anxiety disorders. In a large recent controlled study in London and Toronto, of agoraphobia with panic, high doses of benzodiazepines interfered with exposure in the long-term, and should therefore be avoided. In contrast, in additional work, antidepressants did not interfere with exposure and indeed could enhance it when depression complicated the phobia/panic or obsessive-compulsive problem. Moreover, a variety of antidepressants can be used in such cases as no particular class is yet known to be specific to any given anxiety syndrome.

It is good news that with relatively little help clinicians can learn to give successful behavioural treatment for straightforward clinical problems within a few weeks, and for more difficult cases within a few months. This volume by Drs Stern and Drummond is a fine self-help guide for clinicians who want to learn how to do this.

Preface

The writing of this book grew from regular meetings we have had in which we shared clinical experiences. Most of the cases described are those where we have felt a useful teaching point could be made to illustrate important theoretical developments. We have also argued over the accumulating body of knowledge in the field, and this meant that many drafts were made of each case illustration, so we would have exhausted most typists. Fortunately word-processor technology was available. In consequence, we expect that in the final product it is difficult to identify an author in any chapter. The cases themselves come from an accumulation of many years of clinical experience. In each case we have taken pains to change enough biographical detail to avoid the patient being recognised.

One afternoon the authors happened to be discussing the problems of teaching behavioural and cognitive therapy. Our conversation took the following line: there is no shortage of major textbooks describing the research findings. There are monographs covering a limited area of the field, and multi-authored books that cover a wide area but with no uniformity or consistency. One of us (RS) had published *Behavioural Techniques* in 1978 and that was clearly out of date, and so the idea formulated in both our heads of collaborating in a text to describe the practice of behavioural and cognitive psychotherapy. The book is deliberately aimed at the clinician; so there is minimal reference to the scientific literature.

The book is written for the professional who wants to learn the therapeutic skills in this area. It is not meant to be sufficient in itself to enable one to become a competent therapist, nor is it meant for patients. The professional who uses this volume will need also to receive expert supervision, and will also need to read more widely in the therapeutic literature, and he is so directed at appropriate places in the text.

This is perhaps the place to mention the question of 'sexist' language. In the above sentence the word *he* could have been replaced by *she*, and throughout the text where we use masculine pronouns (or feminine ones) we could have used feminine (or masculine ones).

The general plan of the book has been to begin with some case vignettes to give the overall indications for the therapeutic methods which are then described in the rest of the book. The second chapter takes the reader through our particular ideas on assessment as to suitability for treatment. We then describe some of the more straightforward exposure techniques in chapter 3, going on to apply these to obsessive-compulsive disorder in chapter 4. Self-exposure methods are explained in chapter 5, and then the book proceeds through the wide variety of clinical areas where we consider behavioural and cognitive therapies can be applied. Just how wide we feel this application is can be seen by perusing the contents list: it is no longer narrowed to phobic and obsessive-compulsive disorders, but spans the range of major psychiatric disorders including the problems of depression, the chronic patient, marital and sexual dysfunction. These and other subjects are covered through chapter 6 to 12. In chapter 13 we address the application of these principals to medicine, and then in chapter 14 devote a chapter to the role of medication combined with behavioural and cognitive therapy.

The general principal is that the easier and more straightforward techniques are described earlier in the book, and more difficult cognitive approaches are dealt with at later stages. Within each chapter the standard format is that a method is introduced, a case is described as an example of how to apply the method in some detail, and where necessary the troubleshooting approaches are described and well-known pitfalls are pointed out. Research evidence is not gone into in any detail, as this is best reviewed in other books, but each chapter ends with a summary of the main teaching points that have been made.

We hope that the illustrations by Mandy Assin enliven our text, and we wish to thank her. Many a drawing was done several times, or discarded for the final version, particularly where the authors disagreed. On the whole we did agree that *each picture is worth a thousand words*, and we felt Mandy helped us greatly to make teaching points. Professor Isaac Marks made some helpful comments on the manuscript. Susan Stern read and made valuable contributions to chapter 12, and David Stern re-drew Fig. 2.5.

R.S.
L.D.

London

Acknowledgements

We would like to thank the following for permission to reproduce copyright material: Academic Press for the case history of a dog phobic patient in chapter 3, reprinted from *Behavioural Techniques* (1978); Butterworths Press for the Fear Questionnaire, Compulsive Checklist and Social Situations Questionnaire from *Behavioural Psychotherapy* (1986) by I. M. Marks. The Fear Questionnaire also has the permission of Pergamon Press as it appeared in *Behaviour Research and Therapy*, (1979) by I. M. Marks & A. M. Mathews.

Glossary

activity schedule	a technique where a patient is encouraged to gradually increase his or her daily activity. Most commonly used in treatment of depression to increase feelings of coping and mastery.
agoraphobia	irrational fear of going out alone, particularly into crowded places, including public transport.
anxiety management training	a group of techniques including the use of cue cards and of relaxation, used to treat non-phobic anxiety.
arbitrary inference	a term from Beck's cognitive therapy for depression where a patient jumps to a conclusion without weighing up the evidence or considering alternatives.
attribution effect	an assignment of a cause for an event, and can often be a target in cognitive therapy.
aversion therapy	a behavioural therapy that tries to change unwanted behaviour by pairing that behaviour with aversive consequences.
awareness training	a procedure which teaches patients to be aware when they are indulging in problematic habits or behaviours. It is part of habit reversal techniques.
BASIC ID	a mnemonic representing the major headings described by Lazarus for a behavioural assessment (behaviour, affect, sensations, imagery, cognition, interpersonal relationships, drugs).
behavioural exchange therapy	a term used in behavioural marital therapy where a couple make an agreement to each change a specifically designated piece of behaviour, on condition that their partner does likewise.
behavioural experiment	a test of behaviour, e.g. a patient who cannot go outside the house would be asked to go outside if they could and report what happened.
behavioural medicine	the application of behavioural and cognitive therapy to medicine. It includes the management of conditions subsumed under psychosomatic medicine, hypochondriasis and illness behaviour.
behavioural psychotherapy	a group of treatments with the central hypothesis that psychological distress results from learned behaviour, and can therefore be unlearned.
bridge manoeuvre	a technique in sex therapy whereby penetration is commenced immediately prior to orgasmic inevitability, and then penetration is gradually introduced earlier in the arousal chain.
catastrophising negative automatic thoughts	thoughts which are out of proportion to the evidence, e.g. a patient who feels that as a neighbour failed to greet him, the neighbour hated him.
coaching	a technique used in training chronic patients with basic life skills, by asking them to repeat the activity and providing feedback.

cognitive therapy	used in the treatment of depression and non-phobic anxiety. In depression the goal is to change the cognitive triad, and in non-phobic anxiety to change the negative predictions.
cognitive triad	a group of cognitions described by Beck, that occur in depressed patients. They include (1) negative thoughts about the self, (2) negative thoughts about ongoing experience, and (3) negative thoughts about the future.
cognitive-expectancy techniques	techniques used in the cognitive therapy of depression using the learned helplessness model. When patients fail and make internal explanations for their failure, passivity appears and self esteem drops. Therapy is directed at altering these expectations.
collaborative empiricism	a term used in Beck's cognitive therapy whereby the therapist works with the patient to test hypotheses, and challenge faulty thinking (see empiricism).
communication skills training	a term used in behavioural marital therapy, although it can be applied to other groups of people, whereby the therapist asks the couple to talk to each other to identify any faulty communication patterns. These faulty communication patterns are then demonstrated to the couple. Alternative ways of communication are then suggested to the couple who are encouraged to practise these, often using role-play in the first instance. Feedback on progress is given.
competing response practice	this involves asking the patient to perform a competing behaviour when they have the urge to perform a problematic habit or behaviour. It is part of habit reversal techniques.
covert sensitisation	a form of aversion treatment in which a patient is taught to pair the image of an aversive event with the undesirable behaviour and thus reduce the frequency of this behaviour.
criticism	see expressed emotion. The term is used here to denote high levels of derogatory or disapproving behaviour on the part of relatives of a schizophrenic patient.
empiricism	a school of philosophy that states that all that people are and all that they know are the result of experiences.
expressed emotion (EE)	a term used to describe family interaction style with a schizophrenic patient, and shown to be an important factor in the relapse rate. It has two components: over-involvement and criticism.
flooding	a term, now superseded by exposure, describing a treatment whereby a fearful patient is rapidly exposed to the situations or objects most feared for an extended period of time.
generalisation training	a technique whereby the patient is taught to perform competing response practice in their everyday life without attracting attention from others. It is part of habit reversal techniques.
graduated exposure	a treatment whereby the patient is exposed to the feared situations or objects gradually and systematically, until habituation occurs.
guided mourning	a technique used to help patients cope with bereavement, whereby the patient is encouraged to face up to the situation of loss. The person with abnormal grief is equated to the phobic patient as the patient is avoiding all cues concerning the loss of their loved one. Guided mourning is thus a form of exposure therapy.
habit control motivation	a technique whereby the patient is helped to be more aware of the detrimental effects of their problematic habit or behaviour. It is part of habit reversal techniques.

habit reversal	a treatment that teaches the patient to perform an activity which is antagonistic to the undesired behaviour. It consists of 4 techniques: awareness training, competing response practice, habit control motivation and generalisation training.
habituation treatment	a treatment where repeated prolonged exposure to either a thought or to a situation is carried out.
illness behaviour	this is where psychological factors are thought to be the reason for the maintenance of the behaviour which then manifests as illness.
in vivo **exposure**	a treatment involving the patient facing up to a feared situation or object in real life until anxiety reduces.
Kegel's exercises	these involve contractions and relaxation of the pubococcygeus muscles, and are part of the therapy for vaginismus.
learned helplessness	a condition characterised by an expectation that bad events will occur, and nothing can be done to prevent their occurrence. It results in passivity, cognitive deficits, and other symptoms similar to depression.
magnification	a term from Beck's cognitive therapy for depression where a patient sees small events out of proportion – making a mountain out of a molehill.
mass practice	a technique where the patient is asked to repeatedly perform the unwanted behaviour with the aim of increasing control and reducing the rewarding aspects of the behaviour.
modelling	a treatment which involves demonstrating behaviour that the patient should perform.
negative automatic thoughts	involuntary thoughts of a pessimistic or negative nature that enter a person's mind, in response to specific external or internal events.
negative reinforcement	the removal of an aversive event after a specific response is obtained, i.e. aversive relief. Only of historical interest.
non-contingent positive regard	a term used to describe a warm and caring atmosphere which is not dependent on the patient's actions. It is the best environment in which to introduce a reinforcement programme.
operant conditioning	a term from animal psychology where an animal is trained to perform some instrumental response in order to escape punishment or gain reward. When applied to therapy with patients it involves the use of rewards and punishments.
orgasmic reconditioning	a treatment where the patient's undesirable sexual fantasies are gradually replaced with desirable ones, initially during masturbation.
overgeneralisation	a term from Beck's cognitive therapy for depression where patient has a single experience, e.g. of failure, and concludes that all subsequent experiences will be similar, despite evidence to the contrary.
overgeneralising negative automatic thoughts	are thoughts in which a small piece of evidence is used to generalise to the whole population, e.g. a patient who feels one person does not like them may decide that the whole world is against them.
over-involvement	see expressed emotion. The term is used here to mean overprotective or overconcerned behaviour on the part of relatives of a schizophrenic patient.
over-learning	the technique whereby patients are asked to repeat a desired response or behaviour repeatedly and long after they have learned it. The aim is to ensure that the desired response is 'second nature'.

paradoxical intention	a technique in which the patient is asked to bring on or even exaggerate a symptom in order to face anxiety or overcome a difficulty. He may even be instructed to refrain from something he wishes to achieve, e.g. sexual intercourse. Also known as *logotherapy*.
positive reinforcement	an event which when made contingent on a response, increases its probability.
Premack's principle	high-frequency preferred activity can be used to reinforce lower frequency activity.
primary impairments	a term applied to schizophrenia to denote the main psychiatric symptoms, e.g. auditory hallucinations.
punishment	an unpleasant event which aims to reduce the preceding behaviour.
rational emotive therapy	a therapy where the therapist challenges the irrational beliefs of the patient, and encourages him to engage in behaviour to counteract the irrational beliefs.
response cost	a technique sometimes used in reinforcement programmes where a patient is asked to perform an unpleasant task or behaviour after the unwanted target behaviour, e.g. asking a patient to contribute to their least favourite charity after they had used a swear word.
role reversal	part of role play procedure, where the patient and therapist pretend to be each other to rehearse changes in behaviour or attitude.
satiation therapy	a treatment for obsessive thoughts, whereby the patient is asked to think the thoughts in an exaggerated way for prolonged periods without interruption.
secondary handicaps	a term applied to schizophrenia to denote adverse personal reactions as a consequence of having been psychiatrically ill.
selective abstraction	a term from Beck's cognitive therapy for depression where a patient pays exclusive attention to the wrong cues.
self-imposed response prevention	a component in the treatment of obsessive-compulsive disorder whereby the patient is asked not to ritualise, despite the fact that this may make him anxious or upset.
self-exposure	a treatment whereby the patient, deliberately faces a feared situation.
sensate focus	a technique in sex therapy which begins with non-genital erotic activity, and proceeds to genital play without intercourse. A major role of non-genital and genital sensate focus is to open up sensual communication. It also encourages the couple to enjoy the sensations of closeness without the performance demands of sexual intercourse.
state-dependent learning	this occurs when learning takes place under the influence of a drug, and this learning does not transfer to the non-drug state, and this is known to occur with a number of drugs including alcohol.
stimulus control techniques	a number of procedures in which the patient is taught to control his or her reactions to certain stimuli, e.g. to avoid linking a post-prandial cup of coffee with a cigarette.
stress immunisation	these approaches involve a discussion of stress reactions, rehearsing coping skills, and testing these skills under actual stressful condition.
systematic desensitisation	a technique now only of historical importance, whereby deep muscular relaxation is paired with very gradually increasing anxiety-evoking situations, which may be real or imagined.

tertiary handicaps   a term applied to schizophrenia consisting of social disablements which are either a consequence of the disturbance, or reflect pre-existing factors of deprivation and disadvantage.

thought-stopping   a treatment for obsessive thoughts which involves training the patient to interrupt the thoughts by providing a disruptive external stimulus, which then becomes a self-invoked internal stimulus.

timeout   a form of punishment which involves removal from positive reinforcement for a specified time, usually about 2 minutes.

tolerance   means that increasingly larger amounts of medication have to be given to produce the same effect, and is a very real danger with the benzodiazepine group of drugs.

treatment contract   a procedure where the therapist and patient agree to specify the conditions of treatment in the form of a contract. These are usually written down and signed by both therapist and patient.

1 *Introduction*

Agoraphobia
Sheila said,

Talk about being housebound isn't the half of it, I'm a prisoner who can't go beyond the front gate, I have to ask my friend to collect the kids from school, my husband has to do all the shopping, and I can't go anywhere unless he drives me. It's been like this for three years, ever since I had young George, and the doctor said the pills would help, and I've had the group therapy, but it's all no use . . . do you think *anything* can help at all?

Fear of flying
Adrian was desperate to have help, quickly, for his problem:

If they find out at work that I cannot travel by airplane I will lose my job. The Valium my GP prescribed is no use at all, and if they discover the only way is for me to become paralytic with alcohol then I will be in trouble.

He worked as a civil engineer, had been promoted at work, and needed to make frequent visits to Holland for meetings with clients.

Obsessional rituals
Harriette kept breaking off from her story to ask 'Do you think behaviour therapy can do anything for me?' She was a 35-year-old housewife, severely disabled by not being able to touch her children, her husband, or anything belonging to them. She had developed ideas that the environment had to be kept *sterile* after her first child was born 13 years earlier. She completely avoided dustbins and rubbish bins, and anything that had been in contact with them:

I know these ideas are completely silly but I just can't stop myself. There are also some most embarrassing habits that I feel too disgusted to talk about until I get to know you better . . .

Obsessional ruminations
As he walked along the street John would think 'I know I'm accountable for everything'. He meant by this that if he should witness a car accident while walking along, he *himself* would in some way be the cause of that

1

accident. He knew really that this could not be the case: 'It's an absurd idea, which I try to stop coming, but just can't do it, this idea is stupid but it upsets me, and stops me leading a normal life'. This obsessional rumination was making him depressed, and he feared that he might be going mad.

Social phobia

Jeffrey was hiding beneath a newspaper in the waiting room and when called for his appointment did not even look up. In a barely audible voice he said,

I can never look people in the eye when talking to them and this has made me more and more of a loner. I become hopelessly flustered in female company, especially if the girl is at all attractive. These days I just bury myself in the books in the library where I work, and at lunch time eat my sandwiches all alone.

Sexual dysfunction

Mr and Mrs P. had lived together for 18 months but never achieved sexual intercourse. Mrs P. said 'I think it's his problem as he always loses his erection', but her husband said 'There's no way I can please her, she just gets angrier each time we try, which makes things worse.' It soon became clear that their non-consummation was not due to either one of the partners alone, but faulty technique that had become a fixed behavioural repertoire built up over the months.

Sexual deviation

'Being an ex police officer myself I know what would happen if I were caught . . .' began a 55-year-old man. 'It's just that I get this urge to do it and a tremendous feeling of excitement just before that makes me want to keep on doing it. I feel terrible afterwards and if I get caught again I know it means prison'. He then described how he would wait in a public park for a certain type of woman to appear. He would then stand up and lower his trousers, afterwards feeling very guilty. A previous conviction had focused his mind on the need for treatment.

Illness behaviour

Jill was lying in bed moaning and through her sobs said 'I've never been so bad, you have got to give me some tablets to help, I don't want my husband to lose his job but I can't cope without him here all the time'. She then went on to describe multiple pains in various parts of her body for which she had undergone extensive tests, but nothing organic had been discovered. Her GP was losing patience with her as he was called to visit her several times each week, although on each occasion he was convinced she could have got to the surgery and she always 'recovered' when he reassured her.

Depressive symptoms

Depression has been called the 'common cold of psychopathology'.

Not all symptoms of depression are amenable to behavioural techniques, but when they are, cognitive behavioural approaches are used. Jane said,

I'm a complete failure in everything I do. I'm stuck here in this house with two young children, totally controlled by the situation, and can't do anything I want to. I'm bad tempered with the children, can't cook a decent meal or think of anything to say when my husband gets home from work.'

Cognitive therapy provides a way to help Jane examine the way she looks at her world, and to help her see that she is not really bad at everything. It also uses task-setting to reinforce positive behaviour.

Summary

Several distinct types of problem have been described in vignettes to illustrate *some* of the main indications for **behavioural psychotherapy**, and to whet the reader's appetite to explore the field of behaviour therapy. What do these cases have in common? They all have problems from which treatment goals can be derived, and patients could all agree with the therapist on what these goals might be. In addition they were motivated to lose their symptoms and had something to gain by so doing. By the end of this book the reader should have an understanding of how to set up treatment goals and how to treat the kind of cases described. In all the cases problem behaviour could be measured. Self-recording provides a method of feedback to the patient of his own progress, and allows the therapist to assess change over time. It would not be enough, however, to ask the patient with obsessional rituals how anxious she was feeling if she was made to touch a dustbin. The question was put this way 'How anxious would you feel as measured on a scale where 0 equals no anxiety, and 8 means that you are extremely panicky?' With a little practice it became easy for her to report her anxiety on this scale. All the examples given, except the last, were of problem behaviour that could be observed. In the case involving cognitive therapy for depression the patient's faulty constructs are not, of course, directly observable, but attitudes and depression can be measured.

The plan of this book is to begin with the easier techniques, and work up to the cognitive therapies, and so the logical place to start is with exposure techniques for phobic disorders. Before that it is useful to review the history of behaviour therapy to show how ideas behind behaviour therapy have evolved.

History of behavioural psychotherapy

Behavioural psychotherapy principles go back to earliest times, and can be illustrated by a quotation from John Locke (1693) 'If your child shrieks and runs away at the sight of a frog let another catch it and lay it down a good distance from him: at first accustom him to look upon it; when he can do that to come nearer to it and see it leap without emotion; then to touch it lightly when it is held fast in another's hand; and so on until he can come to handle it as confidently as a butterfly or a sparrow'. (This quotation is cited by Marks, I. M., 1987.) Similar principles were used by a French psychologist, Pierre Janet, to treat a patient with obsessional rituals (1903) and are clearly described in the following quotation:

> The person who assists in the performance of these actions, has a very complicated part to play. He must aid in the performance of the action without actually doing it himself, although the latter would be very much easier; and he must do his utmost to conceal his own contribution to the action, for it is essential that the patient should feel he does the action himself and does it unaided. *The guide has chosen the action, has overcome the patient's hesitations, and has taken the responsibility . . . by continual repetition to perform the action; by words of encouragement at every sign of success however insignificant, for encouragement will make the patient realise these little successes, and will stimulate him with the hope aroused by glimpses of greater successes in the future.* [italic represents this author's emphasis]

Despite these clear examples of behavioural principals, behavioural psychotherapy was not actually defined as a discipline until the 1950s and a useful definition was provided by Meyer & Chesser (1970):

> Behaviour therapy aims to modify current symptoms and focuses attention on their behavioural manifestations in terms of observable responses. The techniques used are based on a variety of learning principles. Although behaviour therapists adopt a developmental approach to the genesis of symptoms, they do not think it is always necessary to unravel their origin and subsequent development.

In the early 1950s, Wolpe was popularising treatment along these lines in the USA. The main technique then was **systematic desensitisation** (SD), based on the principle that: 'if a response antagonistic to anxiety can be made to occur in the presence of anxiety-evoking stimuli so that it is accompanied by a complete or partial suppression of the anxiety response, the bond between these stimuli and their anxiety responses will be weakened'.

Wolpe took over Sherrington's concept of reciprocal inhibition which had been developed to explain the neurophysiology of flexion and extension of a joint (Wolpe, 1958). Sherrington stated that if a flexor muscle contracts, the opposing extensor muscle must be inhibited from contracting at the same time. Wolpe thought that if a person was made to relax during gradual exposure to a fearful stimulus, he could *not* experience fear at the same time, because this fear would be 'reciprocally inhibited'.

There have been a large number of studies on SD, notably that by Gelder *et al.* (1967) where SD was compared with individual psychotherapy and with group psychotherapy, in patients with phobic disorders. SD was consistently better than either of these forms of psychotherapy. Despite its effectiveness SD was a slow and time-consuming treatment which stimulated a search for a quicker and more effective approach.

The result was *in-vivo* **exposure** methods – originally called **flooding** (Stampfl & Levis, 1967). The term flooding has now been largely dropped. *In vivo* exposure methods were pioneered with specific phobias (e.g. Watson & Marks, 1971) and caused quite a sensation when first reported. A variety of specific phobics were treated with rapid exposure in real life with great success. Fears by some therapists that anxious patients would be made worse and other symptoms would appear proved unfounded. The great success of these techniques was also criticised because they had not yet been used for the commonest phobia: **agoraphobia**.

Studies of exposure treatment for agoraphobia were then carried out, for example Mathews *et. al.* (1976), and the treatment was found to be effective. From 1970 to 1980 exposure treatments for agoraphobia were refined and crucial treatment factors were isolated. For example the importance of the duration of exposure in the treatment of agoraphobia was discovered (Stern & Marks, 1973) *In vivo* exposure was found to be more effective than imaginal flooding (Emmelkamp & Wessels, 1975).

There followed a series of studies using sedative drugs to reduce anxiety during exposure. For example, Hafner & Marks (1976) compared diazepam and a placebo in treating agoraphobia. They found that if exposure is kept constant, anxiety is of little significance and the only value of diazepam may be to facilitate exposure. Similarly propranolol was investigated and found to confer little advantage (Ullrich *et al.*, 1975).

Antidepressant drugs have also been used with behaviour therapy to improve the results. Klein (1964) put forward the theory that the central symptom of agoraphobia is panic which is improved by imipramine, so it is claimed. The large literature on the use of antidepressant drugs in agoraphobia is reviewed elsewhere (Marks, 1987).

Over the next few years refinement of psychological treatment factors in agoraphobia continued. It was thought that if treatment could be done in groups it would be more cost effective. Hand *et al* (1974) compared *structured* with *unstructured* groups, and found progress was greater in the structured group. Only the structured group continued to improve after treatment through to three-month follow-up. Group exposure required less professional time and so was an advance in treatment. However, in practice it is often difficult to get a group of similar phobic patients together at the same time and the progress of the group as a whole is linked to the speed of progress of the slowest member.

Another area of investigation was into marital and family factors in the treatment of agoraphobia. Hafner (1977) suggested that since marital dissatisfaction before treatment is related to a poor therapeutic response, a causal relationship must exist between marital state and agoraphobia. Even if confirmed, such data are open to alternative explanations, for example, that both marital dissatisfaction and treatment response are causally related to a third variable, such as general anxiety or to high levels of neuroticism. The existing evidence is inadequate to support a definite conclusion.

Arrindell & Emmelkamp (1986) studied the quality of the marriages of agoraphobic patients. They found that agoraphobic patients and their spouses were more comparable to happily married couples than to maritally distressed couples.

Aside from work with families and spouses of phobic patients, the other development has been the use of self-exposure home-based treatments. This has resulted in a great diminution of therapist time. Marks *et al*. (1983) showed that brief therapist aided exposure was a useful adjunct to self-exposure homework instructions, but even self-exposure homework instruction *alone* is a potent treatment for agoraphobia. Experience to date supports the use of this approach, although involvement of family members in the treatment wherever possible is thought to be beneficial.

The treatment of obsessive-compulsive disorder was developed at the same time as that for agoraphobia, and often by the same workers. Marks *et al*. (1975) reported the results over two years of 20 patients with chronic obsessive rituals treated by real life exposure. This treatment was as effective for obsessive rituals as it was for agoraphobia, although in patients with rituals, treatment was often combined with **modelling** and response-prevention. The principles outlined by Pierre Janet were refined in a series of studies over the years (Levy & Meyer, 1971; Rachman *et al*., 1971), until the present time, when a truly effective therapy can now be offered to most patients with compulsive rituals.

Similar optimism is not justified for obsessional patients with ruminations as the main problem, although in this condition such treatments as **thought-stopping** have been advocated. Thought-stopping is described by Wolpe & Lazarus (1966), and is an early example of a treatment aimed at purely controlling thoughts. Recently new techniques have been developed and are described in chapter 4. Cognitive therapy in general is a recent development in behavioural psychotherapy, and can be applied to anxiety and depressive disorders. It is associated with the work of Meichenbaum in Canada and Ellis and Beck in the USA.

According to Meichenbaum the persistence of many disorders is due to the fact that patients engage in unhelpful internal dialogues when faced with stressful situations for example a patient in a train might say to himself 'If this train stops in the tunnel I shall go mad'. Cognitive therapy encourages the patient to change that unhelpful internal dialogue.

The type of cognitive therapy advocated by Ellis (1962) is called **rational emotive therapy** and can be summarised as follows: if a disorder is caused by illogical premises or illogical ideas patients can often be persuaded or *taught* to think more logically and hence overcome the disorder.

According to Beck, the marked mood swings, which are a typical feature of the depressed patient, are brought on by his own, idiosyncratic automatic thoughts. These take the form of negativistic ideas concerning the person in relation to his environment, which have been well rehearsed over a number of years. As with many habits the individual is unaware of his activity. The main aim of Beck's therapy is to help the patient recognise the unhelpful automatic thoughts, and replace them with more coping and appropriate ones. This explanation of depression can be contrasted with the traditional psychiatric view which regards cognitive dysfunction as a symptom of depression rather than its cause.

As well as a treatment for phobias, obsessive-compulsive disorder, and depression, behaviour therapy has been used to treat other disorders as varied and diverse as schizophrenia and marital/sexual dysfunction. Its application to schizophrenia goes back to the 1960s when Ayllon *et al.* applied operant reinforcement principles to produce changes in patients with chronic schizophrenia. Nowadays behavioural psychotherapy is used to counteract the secondary handicaps of schizophrenia and to assist these patients who are discharged from hospital into the community.

In 1970 the pioneering work of Masters & Johnson led to a range of behavioural techniques for sexual dysfunction, which will be described in this book. There remain a number of other conditions where the application of behavioural psychotherapy has been fruitful, for example habit disorders such as tics, and other pathological behaviours. There is a trend now for behavioural psychotherapy to be used for an increasing range of disorders, and much progress has been made since the first tentative exposure techniques, such as systematic desensitisation.

The current situation

The time is now ripe to integrate behavioural and cognitive approaches into one volume in a way that has not been attempted before. The 'pure' behavioural therapists have long maintained that cognitive therapies are unproven, although the evidence for their efficacy continues to build up, especially in the treatment of depression. To our minds it makes sense to incorporate cognitive approaches into behavioural ones, especially where a pure behavioural treatment is not at first effective or where one is lacking – for instance in the treatment of generalised anxiety states. On the other hand, we take an empirical view – exposure therapy is effective in most cases of phobic disorder; so there is really no need to invoke the more time consuming cognitive approaches those trained in a 'pure' cognitive school might advocate.

Many see all cognitive and behavioural treatments as ignoring the complexities of the human relationship, as reductionistic, and too superficial or even debasing. It should, therefore, be stated that you cannot become a cognitive and behavioural therapist just by reading this book. However, you can become reasonably skilled in these methods by reading this book and attending recognised training courses, and building up clinical expertise under supervision. The techniques described are meant to be applied in a sensitive manner in which the therapist acts as 'guide' assisting the patient to overcome difficulties (cf. Pierre Janet, 1925). The treatments are *goal directed* and to this extent are reductionistic, but they are the goals the patient (the consumer of the service) wishes to achieve, and are arrived at by mutual consent. The therapist requires the humility to recognise that he can only achieve limited goals, and these only if the patient works with him. The criticism that cognitive/ behavioural methods are too superficial implies that there are more *underlying* aspects too subtle to be unearthed by these crude methods, and moreover new symptoms waiting to emerge – the so called *symptom substitution theory*. This theory is just not supported by the evidence. As to the criticism that the techniques are debasing: what is actually done is to offer a treatment that aims to provide a set of tools for the patient to be self-reliant. He is given responsibility for the treatment and expected to work at it outside the consultation room. One aim is to create self-reliance and to avoid *dependence* on the therapist, and another is to avoid dependence on medication as discussed in chapter 14.

The indications for behavioural and cognitive therapy were shown at the start of the chapter by a series of case vignettes to illustrate typical cases where behavioural approaches are valuable. These cases include: specific phobias, agoraphobia, social phobia, obsessive-compulsive disorders, sexual dysfunction, sexual deviation and depressive symptoms.

In order to introduce the book, the development of the ideas and concepts of behavioural psychotherapy was given a historical approach, from the early beginnings in the 1950s with techniques like systematic desensitisation, to the latest, as yet not completely proven, cognitive approaches. In the second chapter we present methods of assessment of behavioural problems. Then we describe the techniques of graduated exposure, the various approaches used in obsessive-compulsive disorder, and the value of self exposure techniques. Thereafter, we continue with the application of behavioural techniques to the reduction of undesirable behaviour, social skills training, and marital and sex therapy. We then relate the ways behavioural and cognitive techniques can be used to change behaviour in the chronic patient, in non-phobic anxiety, and also in depression. Finally we consider the role of behavioural medicine, and that of medication.

The book is limited to the area of adult treatment, as the treatment of disorders of childhood is a growing separate sub-speciality with its own literature. Similarly we have deliberately excluded the treatment of mental handicap.

Towards a philosophy

'The initial power of the therapist as a controlling agent arises from the fact that the condition of the patient is aversive and that any relief or promise of relief is therefore positively reinforcing' (Skinner, 1953). These remarks by the author in his controversial book lead us to speculate why therapists have turned to behavioural and cognitive techniques in the first place, and how behavioural and cognitive techniques may differ from those of traditional psychotherapy. In psychotherapy the therapist does not criticise the patient or object to his behaviour in any way. The behavioural therapist will have carefully defined goals and objectives which are agreed upon between patient and therapist, and the therapist may strongly object if treatment contracts are broken.

The reasons for this are to do with a revolution in the theory behind *neurotic* disorders and the failure of traditional theories to solve the problems of therapy. Behavioural and cognitive techniques require drastic retooling for most traditional therapists and it is likely that those older therapists brought up in that way are unlikely to want to change or to be able to change. In considering the emergence of new theories in science Thomas Kuhn (1970) states:

Philosophers of science have repeatedly demonstrated that more than one theoretical construction can always be placed upon a given collection of data. History of science indicates that, particularly in the early stages of development of a new paradigm, it is not even very difficult to invent such alternates. But that invention of alternates is just what scientists seldom undertake except during the pre-paradigm stage of their science's development and at very special occasions during its subsequent evolution. So long as the tools a paradigm supplies continue to prove capable of solving the problems it defines, science moves fastest and penetrates most deeply through confident employment of those tools. The reason is clear. As in manufacture, so in science, retooling is an extravagance to be reserved for the occasion that demands it. The significance of crises is the indication they provide that an occasion for retooling has arrived.

We take the view that the combination of behavioural and cognitive approaches is superior to any other approach to date for the many disorders described in this book. As research proliferates and these therapies continue to be fruitful the numbers of therapists employing these techniques is likely to increase. The research literature is not the main concern of this volume. The main thrust of this book is to provide examples of how the job is to be done. We aim to show simply and clearly: here are your tools.

2 *Assessment*

Many people assume that there is a great mystery to the art of performing a good behavioural and cognitive assessment. In fact, this is far from the truth and any thorough clinician should elicit sufficient information to enable an adequate behavioural and cognitive formulation to be made, and to implement a treatment regime. Following this procedure, measures of the problem are used to gauge the severity and to enable both the therapist and patient to monitor progress, success or failure of the treatment.

To obtain a behavioural and cognitive assessment does, of course, require that the therapist is a skilled interviewer who is familiar with putting people at ease and dealing with patients. As the skills of psychiatric and general psychological interviewing are beyond the scope of this book, any reader who is unsure about this, should not attempt behavioural and cognitive assessment until undergoing a refresher course.

This chapter is divided into four main sections. The first main section concentrates on behavioural and cognitive history taking and assessment, the second on the behavioural and cognitive formulation, the third on the education of the patient and planning treatment and the final section on the use of baseline and successive measures of the problem. As behavioural psychotherapists are made up of professionals from a whole range of mental health care backgrounds it is important that these assessment procedures are used as an *adjunct to* rather than as a replacement for general assessment procedures, any therapist should have a schema in his or her mind for obtaining general information and assessing psychiatric patients. Just because a patient arrives at a clinic, having been referred for behavioural psychotherapy, does not exclude the possibility of other major mental health problems, or even serious physical disorder. One of the authors recently was referred a lady suffering from agoraphobia whose entire symptomatology of tiredness and palpitation on leaving the house was caused by chronic lymphatic leukaemia which had been previously undiagnosed.

The first subsection – *From medical assessment to behavioural and cognitive history* – of the section Behavioural and cognitive history (below), has been written predominantly for readers with a medical background. Non-medical readers may still find this helpful, although they may wish to concentrate on the subsection *Checklists and mnemonics*.

Behavioural and cognitive history
From medical assessment to behavioural and cognitive history

Many readers started clinical training in general medicine and surgery. In the early days of training much emphasis was given to thorough history taking before moving on to examination of the patient. Unfortunately, many people then become confused when dealing with psychiatric patients, and although they may obtain exhaustive details of the patient's family and early history, fail to gain precise descriptions of current symptomatology. For example, one of the preliminary stages in assessing abdominal pain is to obtain the following information (Macleod, 1973):

1   Main site
2   Radiation
3   Character
4   Severity
5   Duration
6   Frequency and periodicity
7   Special times of occurrence
8   Aggravating factors
9   Relieving factors
10 Associated phenomena

These same 10 questions, with some minor variations, can be almost universally applied to any physical or emotional symptom. For example, if a patient presents with a history of episodic panic, the following information should be obtained.

1   Main site – a full description of what the patient means by panic.
2   Radiation – a full description of the thoughts, fears and emotions of the patient at the time of the above symptoms.
3   Character – a full description of every symptom or change which occurs from the onset to termination of the episode.
4   Severity – the severity of each of the above physical and emotional symptoms.
5   Duration – the duration of each of the above physical and emotional symptoms.
6   Frequency and periodicity – how often do these symptoms occur and do they vary in severity?
7   Special times of occurrence – what time of day, when, where and with whom the symptoms occur?
8   Aggravating factors – does anything make the symptoms worse or more likely to occur?

9   Relieving factors – does anything make the symptoms better or less likely to occur?
10   Associated phenomena – Any other symptoms which have occurred? If the answer is affirmative, then repeat the same 10 questions with each of these symptoms.

After obtaining details of the symptoms in this way, it is important to then trace the progress from their onset, with any variations in symptomatology and details of the circumstances and life events which may have occurred at various times throughout the history. This information is vital as it may radically alter the formulation and resultant treatment. For example, a 25 year old woman presented with a two-year history of fear of dirt and germs for fear that she might catch a fatal disease. This fear was accompanied by avoidance of touching anything that had been touched by other people unless using tissues or rubber gloves, and extensive hand-washing and cleaning rituals. Whereas, at first this may have appeared to be a straightforward obsessive-compulsive history which would be best treated by graduated exposure in real life to the feared situation and self-imposed response prevention (see chapter 4), it transpired that these symptoms had all started after the death of her mother from cancer and that she had failed to mourn this death. Treatment with six sessions of guided mourning (see chapter 12) resulted in complete resolution of her symptoms.

Once the full history of presenting complaints has been obtained in this way, the rest of the details of the patient's life history, family history, past medical and psychiatric problems and their treatments, drug history and social circumstances is obtained in the usual way. Although in a behavioural and cognitive assessment much less emphasis is placed on this information than on the presenting complaints, it is foolhardy to miss out this full assessment of the patient, as without making inquiries in all these major areas, important information which may alter the formulation and recommended treatment regime, could be missed.

The next stage is the *mental state examination,* which is followed by sharing the behavioural and cognitive formulation with the patient, educating them about their problem and discussing the suggested treatment before moving on to obtaining baseline measures and planning treatment in more detail with the patient.

The above description of assessment may sound daunting at first sight, however, there are a number of useful mnemonics and checklists which can be used by the therapist to ensure all the vital information is obtained.

Checklists and mnemonics

When assessing a psychiatric symptom or a problem behaviour it is initially useful to think of two mnemonics both remembered by the letters *ABC*:

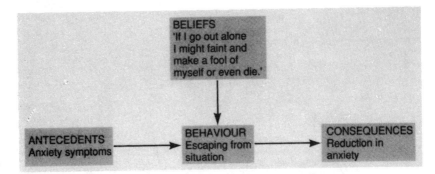

Fig. 2.1. The relationship between antecedents and consequences: example 1.

Antecedents, behaviours and beliefs, and consequences

This mnemonic coined by O'Leary & Wilson (1975), serves to remind the therapist that the antecedents and consequences of a behaviour, as well as the patient's beliefs about it can modify the frequency of the behaviour. Clearly these factors should be examined and form part of the formulation as treatment will usually be geared to modify these.

For example, in the case of June (the agoraphobic patient whose full history is given in chapter 3), the problem could be as stated in Fig. 2.1.

Although similar analysis could be applied to all the case histories given in this book, the case of Flora (chapter 10), also demonstrates the model (see Fig 2.2).

Affect, behaviour and cognition

This mnemonic can not only be used to describe symptoms in a cognitive and behavioural formulation but also can act as a useful model to describe how various treatments alter symptoms (see Fig. 2.3).

This model demonstrates how affect, behaviour and cognition are all interdependent and physical symptoms can alter all three. For example, if we move clockwise around the diagram, and start with affect, it is immediately obvious that how an individual feels affects the way that person thinks. Similarly how someone thinks affects what they do. What someone does has an affect on how they feel. Similarly, the same interrelationships can be seen by moving anticlockwise round the diagram.

If this model is applied to a case which will be described in chapter 3, the outcome is illustrated by Fig. 2.4.

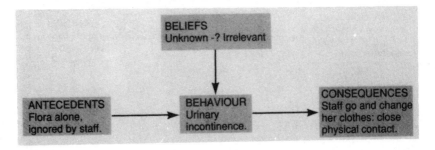

Fig. 2.2. The relationship between antecedents and consequences: example 2.

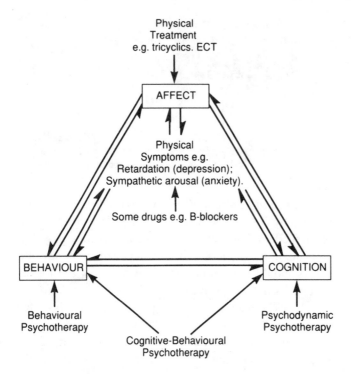

Fig. 2.3. The relationship between therapeutic strategies.

From the example shown in Fig. 2.4, it will be seen that the therapist decided to treat June purely by behavioural psychotherapy. This is because of the interdependent relationship of the various facets of psychiatric symptomatology. Altering June's behaviour was sufficient to alter her negative cognitions, disturbed affect and physical symptoms. This fact is important, as therapists can become prematurely seduced into

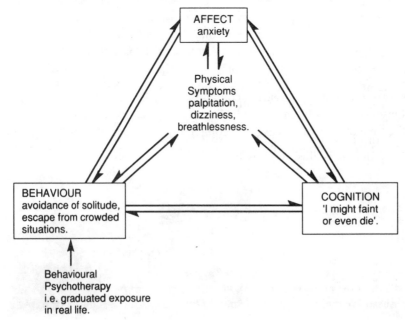

Fig. 2.4. The relationship between behaviour, affect and cognition.

Table 2.1. *Predisposing, precipitating and perpetuating factors: example 1*

Predisposing factors	Inadequate sexual information
	Parental attitude to sex
	School attitude to sex
	Belief that sex was dirty
Precipitating factors	No clear precipitant as life-long problem but perhaps parental disapproval was a factor when patient moved in with Michael
Perpetuating factors	Guilt
	Continued parental disapproval
	Fear of pregnancy
	Michael's attitudes and beliefs

cognitive therapy with a patient with catastrophic cognitions, instead of using the easier and less time-consuming behavioural methods, which are often the most powerful way of altering cognitions.

Predisposing, precipitating and perpetuating factors
Assessment of these factors are a vital part of any behavioural and cognitive assessment, and form a fundamental part of the formulation and treatment planning. In the case history of Lorraine and Michael (see chapter 9), Lorraine's history demonstrates some of these factors (see Table 2.1).

In this example, it is clearly important for the therapist to be sensitive to, and address many of the predisposing and precipitating factors, as well as those which are perpetuating the problem.

However, in the case of Mr. T., the patient who could not reveal his symptoms (chapter 4), it is more difficult to deal with predisposing factors, although they are important information in order to help the patient understand the problem. In this case, a 50-year-old patient had severe obsessive-compulsive contamination fears of 30 years duration. Onset of the problem was following a traumatic sexual relationship. At the time of referral, he avoided completely a number of items to such an extent that he could not even say the words, and he also had extensive washing rituals. See Table 2.2 for an assessment.

Abbreviated assessment or screening

It is sometimes necessary to carry out an abbreviated form of assessment due to lack of time. In these cases it is often useful to remember the plan of behavioural assessment described by Lazarus (1973), as necessary information to devise a behavioural programme. Even a full behavioural assessment can also be performed in this way, although many therapist's

Table 2.2. *Predisposing, precipitating and perpetuating factors: example 2*

Predisposing factors	Family history and presumed genetic predisposition for obsessive-compulsive disorder Obsessive-compulsive mother served as a model Father with obsessional personality demanding high standards High-achieving family
Precipitating factors	Traumatic sexual experience. Perhaps sexual guilt
Perpetuating factors	Total avoidance of 'contamination' cues Extensive rituals prevented any habituation

who already have a standard way of recording information may find this confusing.

Lazarus' scheme can be remembered by the mnemonic **BASIC ID**. This represents the major headings in history-taking thus:

Behaviour
Affect
Sensations
Imagery
Cognition
Interpersonal relationships
Drugs

To illustrate this history-taking schema, the case history of Giles (chapter 6) is described in this format :

Behaviour
Six year history in a 25-year-old man of repeated genital exposure to young women in the public park. The behaviour occurred approximately every four to six weeks, unless a woman had laughed at him or shouted abuse at the previous episode, when he would not repeat the behaviour for several months. The sequence of behaviour commenced by reading pornographic magazines and playing soft seductive music in his bedroom. After 30–60 minutes, he would walk to the park.

At the park he waited in a secluded clump of trees for a suitable 'victim'. The ideal victim was a woman of 16–30 years with blonde hair and alone, although he would sometimes expose himself to a group of women. Once he had seen his target, he would come out from the trees and stand on the footpath exposing his genitals. If he had received a 'preferable' response, he would return to the trees and masturbate to orgasm.

Affect

The initial emotion which precipitated the behaviour was a desire for excitement, which was soon succeeded by a feeling of sexual arousal. This increased as he read his pornographic magazines and played soft music. On walking to the park he would be extremely sexually aroused. At the park, this feeling was accompanied by some exhilaration as he anticipated exposing his genitals but was also excited by the risk of being 'caught'. If his victim demonstrated a desired response, he would feel extremely sexually excited, and would need to masturbate immediately. He would then feel intermittently aroused by the memory of this event for the next four to six weeks until repeating the behaviour. If he received an aversive response, he would immediately experience anger towards the victim, which was superseded within 5–10 minutes by a feeling of humiliation, degradation and inadequacy. Over the succeeding 6–12 weeks, he would continue to feel humiliated, would have a low sex drive and loss of desire to masturbate and would feel miserable and depressed.

Sensations

Preceding the sequence, Giles would feel sexually excited, although erection of the penis did not occur at this stage. This excitement would increase as he remained in his bedroom, and full erection of the penis would generally occur on his way to the park. While waiting for his victim, Giles reported high levels of sexual tension. He frequently believed that his penis would burst unless a suitable victim came by quickly. He was also aware of his heart beating fast, his rapid shallow breathing, and the sensation of his heart beat pounding in his ears. After exposing his genitals, he would generally masturbate to orgasm which was accompanied by a feeling of great release of sexual tension. Thereafter, he generally reported feeling warm, relaxed, satisfied and comfortable as he returned home. On the less frequent occasions when he received his non-desirable response, he would experience a feeling that he described as 'like an icy hand gripping hold of the pit of my stomach and squeezing'. This unpleasant sensation would last for four to five hours, and on occasions had been accompanied by feelings of nausea, and even of vomiting. These sensations would recur over the next 6–12 weeks, whenever he remembered the event which generally occurred approximately six times a day.

Imagery

During early stages of sexual excitement and on walking to the park, Giles would fantasise about having sex with his favourite pornographic idol. Once in the park he would imagine his ideal victim and that she might be so overcome with passion by the sight of his penis that she would immediately make love with him. After exposing himself, if the woman appeared shocked or ran away, he would imagine her returning to have sex with him. This fantasy would be continued during masturbation. Over the following weeks, he would use the image of the woman in his masturbation and would either think of actual events or would imagine that the woman had returned or might return on his next visit to the park to make love with him. If the woman had been abusive or laughed at him, he would have a recurrent image of a school mistress who had taught him in primary school and who had often laughed at him and humiliated him in front of the class. This image combined with the image of the woman in the park would then occur 15–30 times a day and would also occur in his dreams over the next few weeks.

Cognitions

Giles's basic belief and recurrent cognition throughout his behaviour was that, 'Women find the sight of men's genitals highly erotic. If my genitals are attractive enough to a woman, she will be overcome by passion and will make love to me. Even if she does not return, she is likely to become aroused and masturbate as she thinks about the event'. These thoughts occurred throughout the behaviour, and he always expected that, one day, one of his victims would return to have sex with him.

Following an aversive experience he would think, 'That woman must be an old cow, how dare she treat me this way'. After a few minutes when the anger subsided he would think, 'My penis must be abnormal not to arouse that woman. No woman will ever find me attractive but will just laugh at me. I must be the most sexually inadequate man in the world'.

Interpersonal relationships

On examination, Giles appeared a shy and diffident man who avoided eye contact and answered questions in brief, non-discursive replies.

He was the only child of elderly parents and had led an isolated life. His school years had been unhappy as, although an average scholar, he had been bullied by the other children, and had eventually refused to go to school developing symptoms of school phobia and refusal. Referral to the child psychiatric services had not resolved this problem, and he had been taught in a tutorial group with other 'delicate' children.

Thereafter, he had obtained a job as a warehouseman, preferring his solitary life. He had never made any friends at school or in his employment and had never had a girlfriend or any sexual relationship.

Drugs

He was not on any medication at time of referral, but had a previous history of receiving 50 mg chlorpromazine three times daily following release from prison. This had been prescribed by his GP as an attempt to reduce his sexual drive. Giles had stopped this medication after three days as it made him feel drowsy. There was no history of any illicit drug use, and he was a non-smoker who rarely drank alcohol.

The above example demonstrates how a brief behavioural history can be taken. This information would be sufficient for assessing the history of the presenting complaint, and if supported by a full assessment of past history, mental state examination, and physical examination (if indicated), would be sufficient for a full initial assessment of the patient.

Behavioural Formulation

Examples of behavioural formulations will be given throughout this book. However, it is worthwhile asking what is a behavioural formulation and how does it differ from any other type of formulation.

Generally it could be said that a behavioural formulation is a hypothesis about a disorder, behaviour or symptom which attempts to identify any possible predisposing, precipitating and perpetuating factors. It is not carved in tablets of stone and thus, the formulation may alter as treatment progresses and other factors come to light. Usually it is helpful to share the behavioural formulation with the patient; it is often helpful for them to see that their problem, which may have previously seemed insurmountable, can be summarised in a few short sentences and become more manageable. Discussing the formulation with the patient also allows an opportunity for the therapist to ensure that he or she has understood the problem fully, as well as helping patients to feel that the therapist has taken note of them.

A possible behavioural formulation for Gwen (the patient with blood-injury phobia to be described in chapter 3) is as follows:

Although you do not describe any problems with hospital and dental procedures before the age of 14 years, the history of your mother and maternal aunt having similar problems suggests that there may well be some genetic predisposing factors, as well as the fact that you may have learned that these procedures might be accompanied by anxiety and fainting.

After your routine medical examination, you experienced minor symptoms of light-headedness and nausea when told you would need to have a blood sample taken. The fact that the doctor was unsympathetic and the nurse held on to you tightly and roughly would have increased your unpleasant sensations as well as being aversive in their own right. After the procedure, you fainted. You therefore learned to associate visiting doctors with feeling ill and frequently fainting.

Because of your unpleasant experiences, you started to try and reduce the number of visits to the doctor and dentist. Also, you told me that on several occasions you had walked out of a doctors or dentists surgery because you felt so anxious and ill. In fact, both of these moves would serve to strengthen your fear. High anxiety is horrible and therefore a reduction in anxiety is like a reward. In your case, escaping from the situation or avoiding the situation reduced your anxiety. These behaviours were then 'rewarded' by a reduction in anxiety. If you reward any behaviour, you increase the chances of it recurring. Therefore, every time you escaped from or avoided contact with doctors and dentists, you served to increase your fear and strengthen your belief that avoidance and escape were the only way to avoid unpleasant sensations. You, therefore, became increasingly phobic of these situations until the present time.

Similarly, a possible behavioural formulation for the patient who presented with high blood pressure and who is described as 'the man with the impossible life-style' in chapter 13, might be:

You have told me that several of the men in your family have had high blood pressure, so it seems likely that you have a predisposition to this problem. However, we also know that, as well as predisposing factors, most people have precipitating factors resulting in clinical hypertension. You also hinted at another predisposing factor which was that you like to be in control and that you 'do not suffer fools lightly', this tends to suggest that you have what is known as a Type A personality or, in other words, are an ambitious and pressured individual. It is known that people with this type of personality are more likely to suffer from conditions like high blood pressure, but we also know that people with this type of personality can be helped to modify the stress-inducing parts of their personality with good effect on their blood pressure.

It appears that the precipitating events for your hypertension is predominantly your work. You work extremely long hours in a stressful job. No-one can work consistently in a demanding job for 14 hours a day without a break at weekends or holidays, without letting their health suffer. In addition, the recent guilt about your extra-marital relationship and the stress of worrying about the possible effects on your family if this is known to your wife are likely to have increased the chance of a rise in blood pressure.

The chief maintaining factors for your problems are the stress of your work, and the continued fear that your girlfriend may tell your wife about your relationship. Working is, as you clearly said, the most important source of enjoyment to you. A sense of satisfaction with success, the benefits to your family of the good income and the positive feedback which you receive from colleagues all serve to strengthen your contentment with being at work and working. However, it is known that no matter how enjoyable, after a number of hours no-one can continue to work efficiently. The trick may, therefore, be to get you to work efficiently and effectively within more reasonable hours, at the same time as increasing the enjoyment you receive from other areas of your life. Similarly, the situation with your girlfriend appears intolerable. You say you want to end the relationship, but are anxious about this, as she might tell your wife about the relationship. However, you have also thought about telling your wife about it anyway. If you told your wife about the relationship, it sounds as if you would reduce any risk of your girlfriend taking revenge action. Of course, as you said your wife may act adversely, but you felt she would be angry but not leave you. Maybe you have to decide whether this risk is worth the reduction in anxiety.

Education and planning treatment

Behavioural and cognitive therapies differ from most other types of psychiatric treatment, as the aim is nearly always to train the patient to become his or her own therapist. The advantages of this approach are in the cost-efficiency of therapist time, as well as enabling the patient to monitor and implement appropriate action if there is any early signs of relapse. However, this type of approach does mean that more time needs to be spent in the early stages of treatment, in explaining the exact reasons for any suggested remedy.

The case histories described in this book will also demonstrate that a high level of motivation and compliance with therapy is needed in a patient who is often asked to do things that are frightening or aversive to the individual. This compliance can often be dramatically improved by the therapist ensuring that the information given to the patient is honest, accurate and not overly optimistic or even pessimistic. Treatment is usually designed by the patient and therapist together, and not in a traditionally prescriptive manner. In cognitive therapy, the term **collaborative empiricism** has been used to describe the way in which patient and therapist work together to find an answer to the patient's problems (Beck *et al.*, 1979).

Examples of patient education and treatment planning will be seen throughout the book. However, two examples may help to explain this in more detail.

In the case of Gwen (chapter 3), who was mentioned earlier in this chapter with a description of her behavioural formulation, the following information was given to the patient:

The first thing I want to explain to you is about anxiety. Anxiety is an extremely unpleasant experience but it is important to remember that it does no harm to you. People do not die or go mad from anxiety. Secondly, anxiety does reduce if you remain in situations for long enough.

In your case, when in a fear-provoking situation such as visiting a doctor, you initially experience typical symptoms of anxiety such as a pounding heart and feeling shaky. If possible you will try and escape at this time. However, as I have already explained to you, although escaping seems a good idea at the time as it reduces your anxiety, you are teaching yourself that the only way to deal with the situation is to escape from it or to avoid it completely and therefore, each time you escape from a situation, you make the problem worse.

If you do not manage to escape from the situation, another physical mechanism comes into operation and you feel nauseous, dizzy and frequently faint. This is also a part of the anxiety reaction. In the majority of fear-provoking situations, we react with what is known as the fight or flight reaction which we recognise by a rapid heart beat and increased rate of breathing. This reaction is inbuilt and instinctive and prepares our bodies for the physical exertion of either running away or fighting the threat. However, in situations where injury is inevitable, many animals, including ourselves, have an inbuilt reaction which in many ways is opposite to the fight or flight reaction. In this case, the heart slows down, breathing becomes shallow and nausea and vomiting may occur. This reduction in blood flow means that, if injury occurs, you are less likely to bleed to death than if your heart was pumping away at full rate. This is all very well in the wild, but your body is over-sensitive to non life-threatening situations such as a visit to a doctor or dentist.

The way to help is by asking yourself to gradually face up to the things that you fear, and to remain there long enough until your anxiety symptoms subside. This

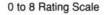

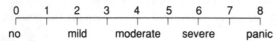

Fig. 2.5. The standard 0–8 rating scale.

often takes between one and two hours. We will now together work out a series of situations which are increasingly difficult, and which you will need to achieve for treatment. For the early exposure sessions at each stage of difficulty, we may have to start with you lying flat to reduce the risk of your fainting. Your anxiety will reduce as you practice each stage, and we will move you gradually into a more upright position. I should also emphasise that, although the treatment sounds difficult, the majority of patients who have this treatment improve. Do you have any questions about anything I have said?

Once the therapist had answered Gwen's questions about anxiety and treatment, the next stage was to establish the overall targets which she wished to achieve by treatment, and then work out a hierarchy of situations of varying difficulty. In order to judge the difficulty of each situation, the therapist asked Gwen to rate her anxiety for each task on a 9 point scale which is used frequently throughout this book and is described fully by Marks (1986). See Fig 2.5.

It is also important not to swamp a patient with too much information, and to ensure that it has been understood. This requires tailoring the information and the vocabulary used to the educational and intellectual level appropriate for each patient.

Finally, patients often forget what is told to them after leaving a professional, and it is useful to provide them with some form of written information to be taken away. This may be in the form of information sheets, or by recommending a particular self-help book (e.g. *Living with Fear* by I.M. Marks, 1978). However, it is also important to give some tailor-made written material of what was discussed in the session and how their problem is viewed. The practice of the authors of this book is to jot down the main points of the behavioural formulation on a piece of paper, and give this along with the diagram of sensitising and habituating exposure (see chapter 3) and the *Three Golden Rules* for exposure to any phobic patient. The latter being written during the interview with the patient, and initially used to illustrate the information given about anxiety.

In the example of Jane, a 31-year-old housewife whose case history is described in chapter 12, and who was treated for depression by cognitive therapy, the following was said:

I understand how very low you have been feeling and you have explained fully to me how recent events have lead up to these feelings. However, it is often the case that it is not events themselves which lead us to feel low but some thoughts which rush into our mind and make us feel miserable.

If I can demonstrate this, I want you to imagine that on my next appointment with you, you did not arrive and did not phone to cancel. Now, imagine that I am prone to get depressed, my thoughts might be something like this:

'She's not arrived, she must think I am a hopeless therapist. Everyone will soon learn about this and realise how useless a therapist I am. I must be a complete failure, no-one could possibly love me. It is pointless continuing to live like this. Now what do you think I would feel like after having thoughts like that?'

Jane replied with a laugh,

Very low and desperate, but that really is not logical because if I had not arrived I might have forgotten the appointment, or written it down wrongly in my diary, or been caught in traffic, or many other things. Also just because one patient missed an appointment does not mean you are a hopeless therapist, and even if you did believe you were a hopeless therapist, it would not mean you were a total failure and no-one could love you.

The therapist answered,

That is right, it does sound silly when stated in this way, but I think we will discover that it is no more irrational than many of the thoughts which run through all of our minds from time to time, and are now contributing to your feeling depressed. These thoughts are called **negative automatic thoughts**, and to illustrate what I mean I would like you to describe to me the last time you had a bout of feeling really low and what was happening at this time.

Jane then described an incident in which she had been sitting having a cup of coffee with a friend. The friend had casually mentioned that her daughter had passed a piano examination recently. Jane found that she felt miserable. The therapist asked her to imagine herself back in that situation, and to repeat out loud the thoughts which went through her mind at that time. The following sequence was obtained:

My daughter has not sat a piano examination yet, she is not good enough. I must be such a hopeless mother that I do not encourage her sufficiently. This pattern will continue throughout her life and she will leave school without qualifications. Once she is unemployed she will blame and hate me. I am no good as a mother, she would be better off living without me.

The therapist then encouraged Jane to examine the evidence which supported and refuted the first of these thoughts: her daughter not sitting a piano examination meant that she was a hopeless mother, who did not encourage her sufficiently. A more rational response that the other woman's child was two years older than her own daughter, her daughter had only been going to piano lessons for three months, and that not everyone was a gifted musician, was then obtained.

Following this, the therapist explained the major thinking errors which people commonly made. These thinking errors are listed fully in Jane's case history in chapter 10. Examples from Jane's own history were used to illustrate these where possible or the therapist gave another example. These thinking errors were then written down for Jane to read at home. She was also asked to fill in the following diary over the next week:

1   Write down each negative thought you have and record the time and place when you have the thought. Put this in the left hand column on a sheet of paper.

2   On the right hand column of the sheet of paper, put down any
      evidence you can think of to contradict the negative thought. If you
      cannot think of any contradictory evidence at this stage, just leave
      the right hand column blank.

In chapter 12 the reader will find a description of how this diary
recording develops into the *two column technique* which is integral to
cognitive therapy of depression. Later on the patient is taught how this is
developed into the *three column technique*, and this is illustrated in Fig.
2.6.

These two examples should give the reader an idea of the level of
information needed to gain a patient's cooperation with treatment. It is
often useful to perform at least some basic measures of the problem at the
same time, as these may help the patient to focus on areas of difficulty
when planning treatment with the therapist.

Measures and rating scales
Are measures really necessary?

Measurement of the problem is taken very seriously in behavioural and
cognitive treatments. Each patient may be considered as their own single-
case experiment. There are several advantages to this type of approach:

1   In initial stages it can encourage the patient to express their own
      targets and goals of treatment, which may prevent the therapist
      fruitlessly trying to pursue a line without the patient's interest.
         An example of this fruitlessness was experienced recently by one
      of the authors, when supervising a trainee psychiatrist in the
      treatment of a patient with agoraphobic and social phobic prob-
      lems. Progress was very slow, despite the trainee spending two to

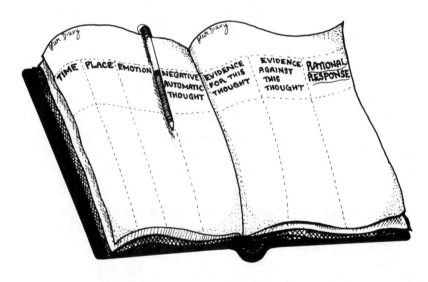

Fig. 2.6. Example of a
thought-diary.

three hours in the supermarket with the patient twice a week. Further questioning of the trainee by the author revealed that the programme had been almost entirely suggested by the doctor, with little input from the patient. Also no measures had been taken as the trainee felt they were superfluous and irrelevant. The author, therefore, instructed the trainee to have another session with the patient in which a full list of measures were completed. This session revealed that the patient had little interest in being able to travel to a supermarket, as she was quite happy for her sister to do the shopping. Thus, she had never performed any of the between-session homework self-exposure suggested by the trainee. Her only target of treatment at the time was to be able to travel on a bus to visit her elderly, frail parents who lived some miles away and whom she had not seen for a year. Changing the treatment programme to tackle this goal greatly improved her motivation, and she achieved her target within three sessions.

2 Measurement allows the patient and the therapist to monitor progress, and to ensure the treatment programme is working. Failure for progress to be made is, therefore recognised early, and the treatment can either be changed or any sticking-points dealt with.

In the example cited above, if the trainee had monitored his patient's progress, he would have realised much sooner that she was failing to make progress, and could thus have saved himself several fruitless hours of his time standing in a supermarket. Also, he would have been able to question the patient earlier and may have discovered her failure to comply with homework tasks and her lack of interest in the target of treatment.

3 The patient may suffer from amnesia about the original problem and overestimate or, more commonly underestimate, the progress or lack of it. This is illustrated by the case history of Mrs. B. a 35-year-old housewife who had a 10 year history of fear of contamination by grease leading to excessive washing and cleaning rituals. At initial assessment, she was housebound, spending her day cleaning the house. Family members were required to strip down to their underwear standing on newspaper at the door before entering the house and changing into non-contaminated clothes. Non-family visitors were not admitted to the house.

Treatment was on an outpatient and domiciliary basis, and consisted of graduated exposure in real life to the feared situation, and self-imposed response prevention. However, Mrs. B.'s high anxiety meant that progress was inevitably slow. After four weeks of therapy she announced, 'Really, you are wasting your time, I am no better and, in fact I think I am even more anxious than before treatment now'. The therapist was able to demonstrate to her how many more things she was doing since the beginning of treatment, and how her anxiety ratings as well as her score on the Compulsion Checklist (see Marks, 1986) all showed a steady improvement. This greatly cheered Mrs. B. who was able to continue treatment feeling encouraged.

4   The therapist may suffer from amnesia about the severity of the patient's presenting problem, and underestimate, or more commonly, overestimate the patient's progress.

This is shown by the case history of Mrs. L., a 45-year-old woman who had suffered from recurrent bouts of depression over the previous 25 years and had received a range of medication. A recent episode of depression had commenced two months earlier, and she had been attending a Consultant Psychiatrist, for the previous six weeks who had prescribed a new antidepressant drug for her. He felt sure that this had had some benefit to her although Mrs. L. denied this.

Whereas some patient's do present with a full range of biological features of depression which resolve completely after a few weeks of appropriate treatment, in the majority it is far more equivocal. A more objective measure such as the quickly completed 13-item short form of the Beck Depression Inventory, BDI (Beck, Rial & Rickels, 1974) would have taken only a matter of a few minutes for the patient to complete at each appointment, and would have provided another and more reliable source of information.

Objectivity and types of measurement

Some forms of measurement are obviously more objective that others. For most clinical cases, the use of self-report or therapist-report questionnaires combined with the patient's, their relatives and the therapist's observations should suffice, but it is useful to consider all types of measure. The following list covers the major categories of measure which are used. It is given in approximate order of increasing objectivity, although this is greatly dependent on the individual involved in the measurement.

1 Self-report

This could just be asking the patient a question like, 'How often do you experience your tic in a day?' which is likely to result in an inaccurate answer but will provide a rough guide to frequency of behaviours. Self-report can be made more useful by asking the patient to fill in a questionnaire containing a number of standard items or by the use of visual analogue scales. Once the patient has completed a questionnaire, an element of self-observation in relation to the rated items often operates, and subsequent ratings are often more reliable than initial self-report ratings.

2 Relative's report
These reports can be useful depending on the relative. They are, however, useful mainly as a confirmation of the patient's report.

3 Self-observation
This requires the patient to monitor and observe their own behaviour over a period of time. The use of a diary is one of the most frequent applications of self-observation.

4 Relative's observation
A relative can also be asked to monitor behaviour in this way as can anyone living in the situation of 'pseudo relative' e.g. nursing staff on a ward.

Impartial professional interview and rating
These measures are frequently used in research and involve a professional person rating the progress who is not involved with, or is blind to the patient's treatment. Frequently, questionnaires are used for this.

Direct observation by role-play (Impartial professional rater)
For some problems, such as anger management training, social skills training and marital communication skills training, role-play can be used to assess the patient's mastery of specific techniques. Objectivity in the use of this as a measure can only be obtained by asking a non-involved suitable professional to rate performance. This could be done either using a one-way screen or, more commonly by recording the role-play on videotape.

Direct observation in vivo
With certain behaviours the therapist can directly observe a patient's progress in real life, for example a patient with obsessive-compulsive contamination fears may have initially been unable to touch a rubbish bin, but during treatment achieves this.

The reliability of these types of measures can be increased by setting up a standard Behavioural Avoidance Test which can be performed by the patient repeatedly during treatment and used to monitor progress. An example of this would be a journey for an agoraphobic patient which might follow a set route, starting with a walk, continuing with a visit to a small shop and buying an item like a newspaper, then moving on to a bus journey, large, busy shops and eventually a train journey. The patient could be asked to return with certain items to prove that they were reporting their actual success accurately. Once again, a 'neutral' professional may be used to assess progress in a Behavioural Avoidance Test.

Direct observation of result of behaviour

The most obvious example of this type of measure is that success or otherwise of a behavioural programme for the treatment of obesity is by weight change. This is an example of one of the most objective measures that can be used. Unfortunately, such objective criteria are rarely available in clinical practice.

Measures and questionnaires

The actual use of different measures and questionnaires is obviously a matter which is subject to a great deal of individual variation, personal preference and personal prejudice. Every psychiatric or psychological journal contains examples of research in which a wide variety of questionnaires have been used to measure a range of parameters.

For someone new to the discipline of cognitive and behavioural psychotherapy, it is best to keep ratings simple, and to become familiar with a few questionnaires. It is best to choose a questionnaire of known reliability and validity wherever possible. It is important to ensure that the measure used will actually measure what you want to measure. This latter statement may sound obvious, but it is common for someone to use a measure of personality trait, for example, when trying to assess a change in the patient's state.

The authors have tended to base the measurement instruments used in the case histories in this book, wherever appropriate, on the system described by Marks (1986). Marks (1986) is worthwhile reading for anyone new to the discipline and to measurement.

Examples of useful measures

Problems and targets

This questionnaire is printed in Marks (1986) and is an extremely useful measure to apply to any patient who is to receive behavioural or cognitive therapy. It should be completed by the therapist in collaboration with the patient.

The first section asks for up to two main problems that the patient wants treated. This is often a useful measure to use before planning treatment with the patient as it gives an idea of how the treatment should be structured. The idea of defining problems can be introduced thus, 'What I want to do now is to try and describe the main problems which you want treated. I have only a small amount of space on this form so we will have to be brief and reduce this to a sentence or two for each problem'. The problem is then written down in a form as close to the patient's own words as possible, although the therapist may have to help the patient by summarising the words or prompting the patient. The patient and the therapist are then both asked to rate how much each problem upsets the patient or interferes with normal activities, on a 9-point scale with 0 = does not and 8 = very severely/continuously (these ratings are done with the therapist blind to the patients ratings and vice versa).

After defining the problems, the patient is asked to devise up to four targets. Targets are clearly defined tasks or items of behaviour which demonstrate improvement and which are considered desirable by the patient. They can be explained to the patient in this way,

What I want us to do now is to define up to four targets for treatment. Targets are specific pieces of behaviour which would be useful for you to achieve and which would demonstrate to yourself and myself that you are improving or are treated when you achieve it. We will define them quite carefully in terms of frequency, duration and situation, so that there is no confusion.

'I want to feel better' is not a good target at all as it is not precisely defined and is open to confusion as to when it is achieved. The patient with moderate depression who gave this answer when asked to define a target of treatment was then told, 'I am sure that is your main aim but that is difficult target to know when it is achieved. What I would prefer is if you could describe to me some of the things you would be able to do regularly if you did feel better, and which you cannot do regularly now'. He then described how he would return to his work full-time, go out with his wife twice weekly for dinner and attend his squash club for a game of squash with a friend at least once a week. The following targets were therefore agreed:

1   To go to work and remain there for eight hours a day, five days a week.
2   To go out to a restaurant in the town centre with my wife twice a week and eat a two or three course meal.
3   To play a full hour-long squash game with one of my friends once a week.

Once obtained, these targets are also rated by the patient and by the therapist (blind to the patient's answer) on a 9-point scale which assesses discomfort and behaviour from 0 = no discomfort or complete success, to 8 = very severe discomfort or no success.

Visual analogue scales or verbal numeric scales
Although this could just consist of a straight line on a piece of paper with no subdivisions, it is often more useful to give a scale on the line. Once a

patient is familiar with rating in this way, it is no longer necessary for him always to have a written scale but verbal ratings can be used to give useful information. As is already clear, the authors generally prefer to use a 9-point scale as favoured by Marks (1986). This can be used to measure anxiety with 0 = no anxiety; 2 = mild anxiety; 4 = moderate anxiety; 6 = severe anxiety and 8 = panic. Similarly using the same gradations, it may be used to measure other factors, including sexual arousal, discomfort, pleasure or indeed almost any emotion that is required. It will already be noticed from the description of the Problem and Target questionnaire that this 9-point scale can be used to measure percentage of success in performing a task.

There is, however, no particular magic in using a 9-point scale and some therapists prefer to use a 10- or 11-point scale. The important point is that the therapist is consistent with the scale, and that both patient and therapist are clear about the meaning of the gradations. Indeed, in the cognitive therapy described by Beck, therapists most usually use a scale from 0 to 100, to ask a patient to rate their strength of belief in a negative automatic thought. This scale with a large number of gradations gives more flexibility for ratings but may, at times, be more confusing to a patient.

Work and home management, social and private leisure activities
This questionnaire described by Marks (1986) is useful for the majority of patients. It consists of four 9-point scales on which the patient is asked to rate how impaired each of various activities is by their problem(s).

Fear questionnaire
This questionnaire which is of known reliability and validity was described by Marks & Mathews (1979). It is useful in assessing phobic patients and gives separate scores for agoraphobia, social phobia, blood-injury phobia and generalised anxiety/depression as well as global phobic scores. (Reprinted in the Appendix 2.)

Compulsion checklist
This has again been subjected to many tests of reliability and validity, and is given in Marks (1986). It is useful only in patients with obsessive-compulsive disorder and is sensitive to change with treatment. (Reprinted in the Appendix 2.)

Obsessive-compulsive discomfort, time, handicap
In order to use this questionnaire (Marks, 1986), the patient and therapist define up to two problems which are then rated in terms of discomfort and time on a 9-point scale.

Beck depression inventory (BDI)

In clinical practice this comes in two main forms, which are useful as either a screening instrument for depression or as a way of assessing depth of depression, or response to treatment. Both forms have been subjected to rigorous tests of reliability and validity.

The short-form of the BDI (Beck *et al.*, 1974) consists of 13-items which are rated by the patient. It has the advantage that being short it can be used as a screening tool for depression in all patients, but also it is useful in severely depressed and retarded individuals who may find a longer questionnaire too much to complete. The authors have also found this a useful questionnaire to give to patients with obsessive-compulsive disorder as they often find a longer questionnaire can take too long if they have the urge to repeatedly check their answers.

An alternative is the 21-item scale (Beck, 1978), which has the convenience of being reprinted in the self-help book recommended for depression (*Coping with Depression* by I. Blackburn, 1987).

Hamilton anxiety scale

This scale is a useful measure for some patients with generalised anxiety disorder, as it is known to detect mostly state rather than trait anxiety, and to be sensitive to change (Hamilton, 1959). One difficulty is that it is scored by a clinician, and its reliability is greater in those who are experienced in its use.

A brief assessment of generalised anxiety and dysphoria can be gauged by the appropriate sections of the fear questionnaire of Marks & Mathews (1979).

This chapter has described some of the measures and rating scales which can be used. Others will be discovered for specific problems, and for many problems it may be useful to tailor-make a rating scale for the patient, and to use this in addition to the standard.

Summary

-   Behavioural and cognitive assessment involves: taking a full behavioural and cognitive history, devising a behavioural and cognitive formulation, education of the patient into the nature of their condition and its treatment, and establishing baseline and subsequent measures of the problem.
-   A good behavioural and cognitive history is similar to a good medical history.
-   Mnemonics can be helpful to ensure all aspects of the history are covered. Examples include: antecedents, behaviour, beliefs and consequences (ABC); affect, behaviour and cognition (ABC); predisposing, precipitating and perpetuating factors (the three Ps);

behaviour, affect, sensations, imagery, cognition, interpersonal relationships and drugs (BASIC ID).

· A behavioural formulation is a hypothesis about a disorder, behaviour or symptom which attempts to identify any possible predisposing, precipitating and perpetuating factors. The formulation may alter as treatment progresses.

· Patient education about their condition and its treatment is a cornerstone of behavioural and cognitive treatments.

· The patient is involved in helping the therapist plan the treatment.

· Measurement of the problem has the advantage of helping the therapist understand what the patient wishes from treatment, and it avoids time-wasting; it also allows both therapist and patient to monitor progress, and to call a halt to ineffective types of therapy. It also ensures that objectivity about progress can be maintained by patient and therapist.

· Measurement of differing levels of objectivity may be needed.

· Rating scales of known reliability and validity are generally preferable in assessing change, but *ad hoc* tailor-made ratings are also useful.

3 *Graduated exposure*

The observation that reliable methods of reducing fear involved exposure to the feared situation led to the development of the exposure principle as the rationale for the success of behavioural treatments for phobic and obsessive-compulsive disorders (Marks, 1973). This development concentrated research and clinical treatment on the important variables of the exposure and the elimination of redundant components, such as relaxation.

The most effective exposure has been shown to be:

> Prolonged rather than short duration (Stern & Marks, 1973)
>
> Real life rather than fantasy exposure (Emmelkamp & Wessels, 1975)
>
> Regularly practised with self-exposure homework tasks (McDonald *et al.*, 1978).

Although the flooding versus desensitisation debate has now sunk into oblivion, there is still concern and confusion in clinical practice about the optimal speed of exposure programmes. Taking a highly anxious patient who has not been out of the house for 20 years onto a train to the January Sales may be effective in dealing with her agoraphobia, but any therapist who adopts such tactics is likely to have a high dropout, and low compliance rate. Also, painstakingly working through a very structured hierarchy with a patient experiencing little or no anxiety at each step is likely to lead to boredom and somnolence in the therapist, and frustration in the patient who sees little improvement after many hours of treatment. It makes sense to tailor the speed of treatment to the needs of individual patients. Some patients are highly anxious and need hours of exposure before they arrive at their treatment goals, whereas others may need little more than the rationale of exposure to enable them to tackle their most feared situations.

Treatment of agoraphobia used to illustrate graduated exposure.

June, a 22-year-old married lady was brought to the clinic by her husband. She had been married for one year and during that time had been unable to go to work because of her fear of travelling alone. Her

33

husband, a security man, needed to work shifts, and was often out all night. On these occasions June would ask her elder, unmarried sister to sleep in the house with her. Once, her husband had been called out unexpectedly at night, June had a panic attack, and had called the GP as she believed she was going to die. Following this episode, they had been referred to the local psychiatric services where the couple had received marital counselling which they felt to have been unhelpful.

First a full history of the problem was obtained. It was found that June, the youngest of a family of two girls and three boys, had always been an anxious and shy person. At the age of 14 years she had been recovering from influenza, and had fainted during morning assembly at school. Following this, she had been unwilling to return to school. After a week at home, she had eventually been persuaded to return, on condition that her elder sister accompanied her to the gates, and met up with her at break and lunch times. Thereafter she was always accompanied on the journey to and from school until she left at age 16 years.

After leaving school she had started work as a typist in an insurance office. This office was close to where her sister worked, and so she always walked to work with her. She avoided travelling on buses or trains for fear that she might faint. Immediately prior to her marriage, she had passed her driving test, but was unable to drive unaccompanied as she feared fainting at the wheel.

She married her childhood sweetheart at age 21 years. Her husband, Barry, was understanding but believed her anxiety problems would improve once she was settled in her own home. They had placed their names on the local authority housing list two years before marriage, and had moved into their flat following the wedding. The flat was five miles away from June's family home, and to get to work she had to catch either a bus or train. She had attempted to get to work on the first day after moving, but had panicked at the bus stop and returned home. Since that time she had remained off work.

After the history was obtained, a working hypothesis for the origin and maintenance of June's symptoms was established. The therapist explained:

Although you have always been a shy and nervous person, it seems that your problems really began after you had fainted at school. This was an unpleasant experience, which you learned to associate with being away from your family. Following this episode, you avoided going anywhere alone, and this strengthened the belief. You never allowed yourself to discover whether or not you could be alone without fainting.

Currently, whenever you are in danger of being alone, you take precautions to prevent this. When you went to the bus stop to go to work, you were tense because of your expectation that something dreadful might happen. Due to your tense state, you began to notice the physical symptoms of your anxiety, for example, your heart pounding and believed that this was evidence that something terrible was about to happen and you might die.

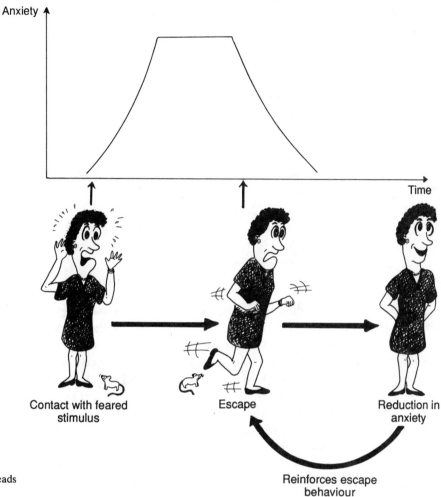

Fig. 3.1. Avoidance leads
to greater avoidance.

Next it was necessary to educate June and Barry about anxiety. Firstly, the possible physical and emotional symptoms of anxiety were explained to them. Then it was described how avoidance of feared situations led to further avoidance, and this was illustrated with a diagram (see Fig. 3.1.).

Secondly, it was explained that during exposure to fear provoking situations, anxiety does eventually reduce, even though this may take up to two hours. Thirdly, that if this exposure exercise is practised regularly, the anxiety experienced gradually reduces in both intensity and duration. To help them remember all this information it was summarised as Three Golden Rules for exposure treatment:

1   Anxiety is unpleasant but it does no harm, i.e. I will not die; go mad or lose control.
2   Anxiety does eventually reduce, i.e. it cannot continue indefinitely, if I continue to face up to the situation.

3   Practice makes perfect, i.e. the more I repeat a particular exposure
       exercise, the easier it becomes.

These rules are illustrated in Fig. 3.2.

Following this explanation of the rationale of exposure treatment, it
was necessary to identify the targets of treatment with the patient herself.
June identified five specific tasks which she would like to be able to
perform by the end of treatment, and which would demonstrate to both
herself and her therapist that she had improved:

1   To drive alone on the motorway to visit an old school friend in
       Camberley.
2   To travel to work alone on the bus during the rush hour.
3   To travel to work alone on the train during the rush hour.
4   To travel alone by bus and underground train into the centre of
       London, and to visit the main shopping areas.
5   To remain in the flat alone overnight while Barry is on a night-shift.

June decided that it would be easiest for her to start by tackling her
problem of walking alone. Barry agreed to be involved in the treatment,
and to act as her co-therapist. As there was insufficient time at this first
meeting for any therapist-aided exposure, June and Barry agreed to start
the programme during the week. Every evening, when Barry returned
from work, they were to go out for a walk. June was to leave first and to
travel along a predetermined route, while Barry was to wait for five
minutes and then follow in her footsteps. They were to take care that the
exposure time was long enough for June's anxiety to reduce (habituation), which usually takes between one to two hours. June was to record
the details of the exposure exercises in a diary, and to also note down her
anxiety levels at the beginning, middle and towards the end of the
exposure task. To introduce some consistency into the anxiety ratings,
she was asked to record the level of anxiety using a 0–8 scale where 0
meant no anxiety and 8, extreme anxiety or panic. This scale is described
in chapter 2. If June found her anxiety levels reducing during the week,
she was to go out for a long walk alone with Barry remaining in the house.

At the second session the following week, June and Barry were
delighted with the progress. June had managed not only to walk alone,
but had even visited the local shops and carried out some shopping while
Barry remained at home. The therapist praised her for this excellent
progress. It was suggested to June that, with her consent, the session
could be used to start tackling bus travel. She agreed, but felt that she
would prefer to start with old-fashioned buses with an open exit rather
than the more difficult driver-only buses with doors that shut. At first,
June asked if Barry could sit next to her, but eventually agreed to sit at the
front of the bus, while Barry and the therapist sat at the back. After a few

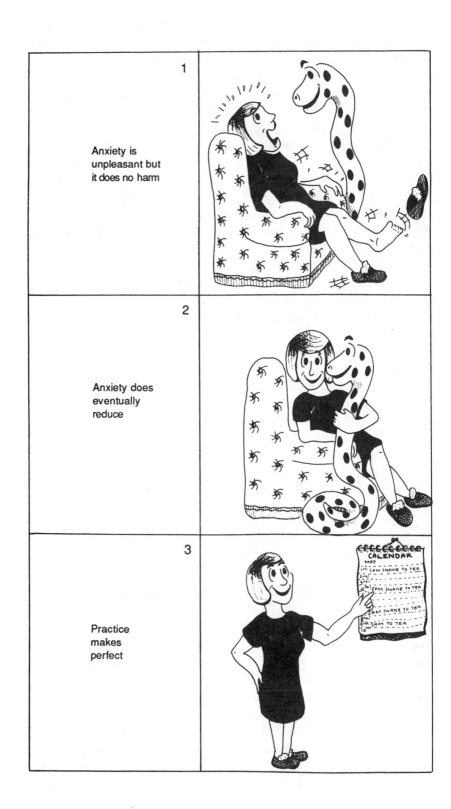

Fig. 3.2. The Three Golden Rules.

minutes, June became very anxious and came to the therapist complaining of symptoms of panic. She was gently reminded that this feeling, although unpleasant, would eventually pass, whereas, if she gave up now, her anxiety might be even worse next time. She returned to her seat and after a further 45 minutes looked much more relaxed and cheerful. At the pre-arranged stop, June, Barry and the therapist left the bus. June was praised by the therapist who said:

'You have done extremely well. Despite feeling panicky you have managed to face up to your fear, and have learned that these frightening and nasty symptoms do eventually reduce'. Following the praise from both the therapist and her husband, June expressed her feeling of delight with her achievement, and requested that she might go alone into a nearby supermarket and buy some shopping, while Barry and the therapist remained outside. She was again praised for this decision, and succeeded in buying a trolley of groceries despite the crowds in the store.

On the return journey, June sat alone upstairs on the bus while her husband and the therapist sat downstairs. Again, she coped excellently, and readily agreed to continue this practice with Barry during the following week. She was to start using driver-only buses once her confidence increased, and to tackle bus travel alone while Barry remained at home.

For the third session, it was arranged that the therapist would meet June alone outside an underground station. Barry was, unfortunately, at work and unable to attend that week. June travelled to the station alone on a bus. During this session exposure to underground travel was performed in a similar way to the session with bus travel. The fourth and fifth sessions were given at the outpatient clinic. June and Barry gradually increased the homework exposure, so that June practised travelling alone to her place of work by bus and train, and was able to return to work before the end of the fifth week. She also travelled up to London alone when Barry was at work. During this time, June began working on her fear of remaining alone in the house overnight. Initially, she stayed alone in the house during the day and evening, and then progressed to remaining alone overnight when she knew that her sister was at home. She was pleased and surprised with herself when she did not feel the need to phone her sister, and felt able to try being alone without taking these precautions. Throughout this time the therapist monitored her progress, praised her for her success, and suggested tasks that she should attempt.

By session six, most of the treatment targets had been achieved, however, driving alone had proved more difficult for her. Barry was concerned that she might become very anxious when driving and 'do something silly', and so had been unwilling to encourage her to practise driving. As June found it easier to drive on quiet roads, the therapist and Barry sat in the car while June drove from the clinic into the country. Again, she found this easier than she had anticipated and agreed that, after 45 minutes of driving, she would stop at a station and leave the therapist and Barry to catch a train while she drove herself back to the clinic. This demonstration proved to both June and Barry that she was able to drive sensibly and safely. Following this session, June continued to practise driving over the next three weeks. Initially, she continued on quiet roads, and then on increasingly busy roads in town. Driving in lines of traffic when she was in the right-hand lane and felt unable to 'escape' were particularly difficult for her, and so she devised some routes which involved doing this. Her confidence increased as she practised, and she began travelling on motorways. Once again, she began by driving on motorways at relatively quiet 'off-peak' times and then progressed to busier times.

Session seven was used to reiterate the principles of treatment, which June had successfully learned and applied. She had achieved all her targets of treatment. The therapist warned her that she would still need to continue practising over the following months. Everyone has good and bad days, weeks or months and the important thing would be for June to continue to face up to difficult situations even during the *bad* times when she felt more anxious. Any periods of illness which restricted her activities may well lead to a slight increase in fear when she returned to normal. Finally, she was congratulated for all her success and hard work. Arrangements were made for her to be reviewed at one, three, six and 12 months to ensure that her gains were maintained.

June's case demonstrates how a young woman with a moderately severe phobia was treated, with the help of her husband and 14 hours of therapist's time over a seven-week period. Some patients, however may require more or less time and not every patient has a helpful and willing spouse, relative or friend who will act as co-therapist.

Case history of flight phobic

Adrian, a 27-year-old unmarried civil engineer, worked for a large successful firm in London. Recently he had been promoted at work, and was asked to take responsibility for a job the firm was to undertake in Holland. This required him frequently visiting Amsterdam for meetings with the clients. Adrian had a four-year history of fear of travelling by plane. He had so far managed to keep his fear secret by arranging meetings for Monday mornings, and then travelling over to Amsterdam by boat and train on Sunday. However, he realised that he would not be able to maintain his pretence for long without being discovered. He was worried that, if his problem was known at work, his future career might be jeopardised as his bosses would think him 'a nervous wreck'.

The onset of Adrian's problem had occurred four years ago, when he was returning to England from a holiday in India. The flight had been particularly turbulent, and he had suddenly remembered some details of a similar aircraft being involved in a crash a few months previously. He had felt anxious and nauseous throughout the remainder of the flight. Since that time, he had felt unable to travel anywhere by plane unless he took diazepam (prescribed by his GP), and alcohol until he had almost total amnesia for the journey. Whereas he had managed to travel in this state in the company of relatives or friends to go on holiday, he realised that he could not do this if travelling to attend a business meeting.

After the history was obtained and he was given the rationale of exposure treatment, the patient agreed to start a programme of self-exposure by visiting the airport every evening and remaining there to watch aircraft take off and land and the passengers checking in their luggage. He was asked to imagine that he was actually about to travel while at the airport and to remain there until his anxiety subsided. It was explained that taking alcohol or tranquillising tablets were forms of avoidance, and so although initially reducing anxiety, in the longer term, they strengthened and increased his fear.

Ten days after this initial assessment, the therapist received a phone call from Adrian who was at the airport. He reported that he had initially felt extremely anxious and nauseous when visiting the airport, but that this had improved as he continued to practise. He had noticed that one of the airlines offered day trips to an unknown destination, and wondered if the therapist would be willing to accompany him on such a flight. The therapist agreed, and a mutually acceptable date was arranged so that Adrian could book the seats.

On the day the flight was arranged, the therapist met Adrian at the airport. He appeared anxious and rated his anxiety as 6 on an 8 point scale. Previously, he said that he would have gone immediately to the bar 'to settle his nerves' when he felt anxious, but managed to remain in the queue to check on to the flight, and then accompanied the therapist to the departure lounge. The destination for the trip was Cologne and Bonn airports, involving just over one hour's flying time, which when considered with the delays and return journey, would allow sufficient time for Adrian's anxiety to reduce.

When the flight was called, Adrian developed symptoms of panic. He appeared flushed, sweaty and tremulous. He said that he felt he had made a mistake, and that he wished to leave the airport, return home and to continue practising the visits to the airport before attempting to fly. The therapist responded by pointing out:

> I can see that you are extremely anxious and realise how unpleasant that must be. However, if you go home now, it will be much more difficult for you the next time you try. Although you feel very anxious now, you will remember that the first time you came to the airport you were also quite panicky. No matter how dreadful you feel now, that feeling will pass as long as you continue.

Following this, Adrian stood still and did not appear to be about to run from the lounge. The therapist noticed that he was breathing very rapidly and felt that this hyperventilation was likely to be contributing to

Adrian's discomfort. Instructions for taking slow deep breaths were given to him in this way:

> I see that you are breathing very rapidly and shallowly. This kind of breathing often makes people feel much worse and adds to their symptoms. What I would like you to do with me now is to place your hand onto your tummy. You should be able to feel your tummy moving in and out if you are breathing correctly using your diaphragm. Now, drop your shoulders down and try and relax them and keep them still – you do not need to use your shoulders if you are breathing correctly. Good, you have done that well. I am now going to count slowly to five several times. I want you to breathe in slowly and feel your tummy push out for the first count to five. Then, I would like you to hold your breath for the next count to five and lastly to breathe out slowly and regularly for the final count to five. We will then repeat this a few times until you can do it on your own.

After a few trials, Adrian had slowed his breathing, and reported that he was feeling a little better. By this time there was an announcement for the remaining passengers to board the aircraft immediately. Adrian agreed to continue and boarded the aeroplane. The flight was moderately turbulent throughout. Adrian reported that he was tempted to have a drink when the air hostess arrived with the bar, but realised that this would worsen his problem. Despite this, he appeared much less anxious by the time he landed in Cologne and Bonn.

For the day trip flights, passengers are asked to leave the aircraft and to enter the arrivals lounge, but not to pass through customs as the return flight boards almost immediately.

On the return flight, Adrian was much more confident. He asked if he could change seats with the therapist to sit next to the window, and look at the clouds and the view. At the time of landing in London, he reported that he was enjoying the flight. Following this therapist-aided session, Adrian arranged to fly to Amsterdam for a business meeting. At six-month post treatment follow-up, he was flying regularly to Europe and recently had booked a holiday in California. He reported that he still found it helpful to avoid alcohol prior to or during a flight as he felt that any feeling of 'light-headedness' increased his anxiety. Adrian's success illustrates how even one session of therapist-aided exposure can effect a significant and lasting change in phobic anxiety. Not all phobias are dealt with so easily and quickly, however.

A more severely disabling phobia which took several months to treat, is now illustrated

Case history of a severe, life-threatening phobia

Gwen, a 35-year-old married woman was referred to the clinic because of her extreme fear of any medical or dental procedures. For years she had avoided any contact with the medical profession, but recently had forced herself to attend her GP because of a marked and sudden abdominal swelling. She had been referred to the local hospital, and had only been able to attend there after taking 40 mg of diazepam to lower her anxiety.

A large ovarian cyst was diagnosed. Her gynaecologist advised that a laparotomy operation was needed. Gwen felt unable to consent to this, and had refused to re-attend the hospital or her GP. Indeed, she was reluctant to come to a psychiatric clinic and would only attend when reassured that the building was separate from the general hospital, and that there would be no medical equipment in the room.

The onset of her fear was at age 14 years when she had been required to give a blood sample following a routine medical examination in school. She felt anxious, nauseous and light-headed. The medical officer had not been sympathetic, and had gruffly told her to 'Pull herself together'. The nurse had then held tightly onto her arm to prevent her from moving. The blood sample had been taken, but she had fainted immediately after the procedure. From that time, she had felt faint whenever visiting her GP or a hospital. The fainting had deteriorated over the years until she avoided these situations. She had painful dental caries as she had avoided attending the dentist for the past 10 years.

The assessment interview was complicated by Gwen's extreme fear. She frequently retched and complained of feeling faint. Much of the interview was performed with Gwen clutching a sick bowl lying flat on the examination couch. Luckily, her husband was able to supply many of the details for her.

As with the previous cases, Gwen and her husband were educated about anxiety and exposure. In addition, it was necessary to explain to them that phobias of blood, injury and medical interventions were often different to other phobias because as well as the anxiety reaction (predominantly mediated by the sympathetic component of the autonomic nervous system), there was additionally a fainting reaction (mediated by the parasympathetic component of the autonomic nervous system), which meant that exposure therapy would be performed with Gwen lying flat at first. As she progressed with exposure and her physiological responses reduced, she would be gradually raised into an upright position. Because Gwen was extremely anxious, it was important to emphasise that nothing would be done without her prior consent, and that the therapist and her husband would not try and trick her in any way. Her husband, Frank, agreed to act as co-therapist.

Gwen's main target was to undergo the necessary laparotomy operation, but her intermediate targets were :

1   To have my blood pressure taken.
2   To visit a hospital ward and remain there for several hours without fainting.
3   To have an injection.
4   To have a blood sample taken.
5   To give a pint of blood at the Blood Transfusion Centre.

The details of Gwen's exposure programme and her homework practice are shown in the Table 3.1.

Table 3.1. *Example of therapist-aided exposure at clinic*

Session no.	Details of exposure	Length of exposure sessions (hours)	Homework tasks
1	Staying in psychiatric clinical environment until anxiety reduces Looking at pictures of blood, injury and medical procedures	2	Visit: Hospital waiting rooms. GP's surgery waiting room Hospital ward Accident and emergency department Looking at medical pictures
2	Applying tourniquet and sphygmomanometer to therapist's, husband's and own arm Using alcohol swab on arm	$1\frac{1}{2}$	Applying tourniquet and alcohol swabs to own arm
3	Examining and handling a variety of needles and syringes	$1\frac{1}{2}$	Handling needles Injecting an orange
4	Watching therapist and husband have subcutaneous and im injections Having subcutaneous injection herself	$2\frac{1}{2}$	Visit general practitioner and receive inoculations required Visit dentist and commence cour of treatment
5	Watching therapist and husband having phlebotomy performed	1	Watch video of therapist undergoing phlebotomy
6 7 8	Having phlebotomy performed	5	Visit GP and have blood sample taken
9	Watching therapist and husband donate blood at Blood Transfusion Service Donate Blood herself	2	Continue some of exercises above
10	Visit gynaecology ward; meet nursing and medical staff Discuss planned operation	3	Admission to hospital for laparotomy

Total therapist-aided exposure = $28\frac{1}{2}$ hours over 10 weeks

This case shows how exposure can sometimes be a slow process with a highly anxious subject, but that ultimately success is achieved. In these cases, it is important to obtain objective measures of anxiety and goals of treatment. Otherwise, the slow but sure progress may have been over-looked by both patient and therapist, who might have abandoned treatment in the belief it was unsuccessful.

The use of modelling

Modelling is a procedure often used to facilitate exposure therapy. In this technique, the therapist models an activity that the patient is afraid to perform and asks the patient then to follow suit (Bandura, 1970). This procedure was combined with exposure in the treatment of the cases presented in this chapter, but is illustrated in a more obvious way in the treatment of a *specific dog phobia*.

The patient was an 18-year-old student teacher who, since childhood, had avoided situations where she might come into contact with dogs. The family protected her in this way and someone always had to check the garden at her home to ensure that no dogs had strayed in before the patient went there. She had to cross the road to avoid dogs and never went into public parks for the same reason. An interesting point in her past history was that her mother remembered that, at age two years, the patient had been frightened by a large dog jumping onto her pram. However, the patient herself had no recollection of this event.

In the first treatment session the patient eventually agreed to remain in the same room as a small dog, if the dog was never closer to her than 12 feet (4 m), and then only if it remained on a leash. The therapist sat down on a chair close to the dog and petted and stroked it while talking to the patient. After about 20 minutes, the patient approached the dog and was able to imitate the therapist's stroking action along the dog's back. In the first session, she could not be persuaded to touch the head of the dog and would not touch it at all unless the therapist kept it on a leash. On leaving the treatment room after this session, the therapist returned to the waiting room with the patient. The patient's aunt who was waiting for her said 'She will never agree to having a dog in the same room'. The patient then related to her aunt what had transpired in the treatment session.

Subsequently four more sessions were required where the emphasis was on modelling to facilitate exposure to the dog: the therapist modelled touching the dog's head, even putting a hand into the dog's mouth. Eventually, the patient was able to follow suit, even when the dog was unleashed.

Part of the treatment involved homework exercises in which she had to visit a friend with a large dog. By the end of treatment she could remain alone with the dog in a friend's room. At follow-up one year later, she was able to visit public parks and had no fears of encountering dogs off the leash.

Summary

- Graduated exposure *in vivo* is effective in the management of phobic anxiety.
- Exposure should be tailored for the individual patient, and should be performed at the maximum speed that he or she can tolerate.
- Realistic treatment targets must be decided with the patient at the commencement of treatment.
- A helpful spouse, relative or friend can often be usefully incorporated in the exposure treatment.
- Homework practice between treatment sessions is vital.
- Modelling can be used to facilitate exposure.
- Education about the rationale of exposure is important, so that the patient can learn to become their own therapist, and deal with any recurrence of fear before deterioration occurs.

4 Treatment of obsessive-compulsive disorders

In the previous chapter we demonstrated the use of graduated, prolonged *in vivo* exposure in the treatment of phobic anxiety. Obsessive-compulsive symptoms often resemble phobias but there are also some important differences as shown in Table 4.1.

At first this may seem a complicated distinction, but some examples will demonstrate the differences. At the end of chapter 3, we related the case history of the student teacher, Julie, who had a fear of dogs. This fear was an example of a specific animal phobia as the fear was purely related to the presence of dogs in her vicinity. Contrast this with the case of Eleanor, who had a 10 year history of fear of contamination by dirt from dog faeces, as she was concerned that she might catch a variety of diseases, which could then be passed on to others and which would result in her feeling responsible for this plague. This problem caused her to avoid any situations where she had seen dogs in the past. Even if she saw a dog through her window she would feel anxious and resort to cleaning rituals. Her anxiety-reducing rituals consisted of stripping off all her clothes which were then considered contaminated and washing these: she would bathe in a set pattern and would repeat this ritual washing in multiples of four which she considered a 'good' number.

In Julie's case she had a classical dog phobia which lead to avoidance of dogs or any situations which reminded her of dogs. Eleanor's problem was different in that her fear was not of dogs themselves, but of the

Table 4.1. *Comparison of obsessive-compulsive disorder (OCD) and phobic disorder*

OCD and Phobias	
Similarities	Differences
1 *Anxiety* accompanies the obsessional thought or ritual	1 In OCD the *fear* is *not* of the situations themselves but of their *consequences*
2 *Avoidance* of situations which provoke thoughts, anxiety or rituals	2 Elaborate *belief systems* develop around the rituals of OCD, but not around phobias

consequences which she thought may result from contact with dogs. Unlike Julie whose anxiety is relieved by escaping from the dog, Eleanor would still remain anxious after the dog had left until she had performed her washing rituals to her satisfaction. The development of *elaborate belief systems* in people with obsessive-compulsive disorders is also demonstrated by Eleanor, who performed her stereotyped washing rituals in multiples of four. However, these belief systems are only part of the phenomena, as people with obsessive-compulsive disorders generally realise that their fears are irrational, and that their ritualistic patterns are unrealistic.

Treatment in both Julie's and Eleanor's cases was similar. Both received graduated prolonged exposure to their feared situation. There was an additional component in Eleanor's treatment because of the rituals. This is called **self-imposed response prevention** or in other words, explaining to the patient the effect of rituals on anxiety and then asking them not to ritualise. In Eleanor's case, after the therapist had taken her history and talked to her about anxiety, the following explanation was given:

When you are in contact with anything which makes you feel 'contaminated', you experience extreme anxiety. A high level of anxiety is uncomfortable, and so being human, you will try to escape or avoid that experience. However, escaping from the situation is not possible if you already feel 'contaminated'. In order to reduce your anxiety you have therefore developed the anxiety reducing rituals of washing in a set pattern in multiples of four. When you perform these rituals, your anxiety reduces.

As high anxiety is uncomfortable, this reduction in anxiety is like a reward. You are therefore rewarding your ritualistic behaviour. If we reward any behaviour then we increase the chance of it recurring in that situation again. For example, if a dog sits up and begs and is rewarded with a chocolate drop, then you increase the chance of it sitting up and begging again.

In the case of obsessional rituals, however, although they reduce anxiety, there are 2 problems:

1   They only reduce anxiety a small amount.
2   The anxiety reduction is short lived and you then have to repeat the ritual.

In practice this means that you are constantly experiencing very high levels of tension and anxiety. I am going to ask you to stop performing any rituals at all. Although this sounds difficult, I think you will soon find that your anxiety eventually reduces much further than when you ritualise. Old habits die hard and you may on occasion, find yourself ritualising. That is fine as long as you stop once you realise and then 'recontaminate' yourself.

The graph shown in Fig. 4.1. was also drawn for Eleanor during this explanation.

Most patients with obsessive-compulsive disorder have the complete syndrome, that is, obsessions *and* compulsions. Some patients have only the ideational component, that is obsessions. A very small percentage of patients have only the motor symptoms, that is compulsions. Many

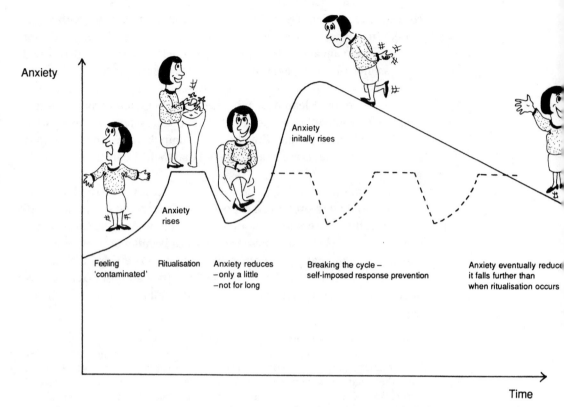

Fig. 4.1. The relationship between anxiety and rituals.

patients only complain about their compulsions but careful questioning often reveals some obsessional ideas as well, although in the very chronic patient, these may have been lost in the distant past.

The basis of treatment for these conditions is *exposure* to the anxiety producing obsessions or the stimuli which produce these thoughts. *Self-imposed response prevention* is additionally used as a way of prolonging exposure.

The application of this rule of exposure and self-imposed response prevention is much simpler in a patient with clear-cut anxiety producing obsessional thoughts *and* anxiety reducing rituals. *Obsessional ruminators* without overt obsessions have traditionally been more difficult to treat (Stern, 1978b). Careful behavioural analysis, however, will often reveal that the patient has two elements to their 'rumination'. Firstly, they will often have an anxiety-provoking obsessional thought which is then followed by an anxiety reducing cognitive ritual. In these cases the same principles of exposure treatment apply. There is a difficulty in producing reliable exposure without the patient automatically 'cancelling' or 'putting the thought right' in his or her head. Recent research has been addressed to this specific problem (Salkovskis, 1985).

A compulsive ritual is defined as a piece of behaviour that the patient feels compelled to carry out despite the recognition of the senselessness of the action. It used to be considered necessary for the patient to have a subjective internal feeling of resistance to the compulsion (Lewis, 1935), but more recent studies have shown that this is not always the case (Stern & Cobb, 1978).

The techniques reported in this chapter are based on numerous controlled trials carried out in Europe and the USA, and are reported in detail by Marks (1987), who states: 'Few improvements are more satisfying for the clinician to see. Treatment can restore normal family life in patients who for a decade or more had hands raw and bleeding from washing all day, would never touch any family member, crippled the family with incessant demands that they wash as well, prevented them from having visitors in the house for years, vetoed family holidays, and caused them to move repeatedly for fear of dirt'.

Early studies implied that 24-hour response prevention was necessary, but recent evidence suggests that shorter sessions are just as good, and it may be possible to obtain good results when the therapist does no more than act as coach to the patient's own homework programme of self-administered exposure plus response prevention (Hoogduin & Hoogduin, 1983; Marks, 1987).

A common compulsive ritual is excessive handwashing:

Treatment of compulsive handwashing linked to a contamination obsession

'I have always been meticulous but recently things have got completely out of hand' said a 52-year-old lady. She went on to describe that five years ago she had started paying excessive detail to her every action, and household chores such as washing and ironing had become so time consuming, because of this attention to detail that she dreaded them. Many rituals centred around dressing herself and personal hygiene: for example when hanging up a dress, she could not do so *without* shaking out the dress six times and then examining it from every corner, which meant the procedure took at least 30 minutes. In addition, if she had touched anything that she considered 'dirty' such as a rubbish bin, or 'smelly' such as an onion, she became very anxious and felt compelled to wash for at least 40 minutes afterwards. 'These rituals are ridiculous, they take up all my time and make life a misery', she said.

She was happily married with two grown-up children. Her husband pointed out that in the last few years the rituals had gradually taken over her life. He was keen to help in any way he could with her treatment, but Mrs. K said she would be too embarrassed to let her husband become involved. Although the involvement of relatives is usually thought to be essential, in this case it was decided to respect her wishes as long as the husband's non-involvement did not impede treatment: he understood never to reassure her that she was *not* contaminated, and never to become involved in the rituals.

Behavioural formulation

THERAPIST: What happens if you touch something dirty or smelly?
PATIENT: I get very anxious, even though I realise there is no logical reason for it.
THERAPIST: And then washing makes you less anxious, and that causes washing to become rewarding behaviour, that is increasingly likely to reoccur, because each time you wash you reward yourself again.
PATIENT: You mean it's like a habit, a kind of ingrained behaviour pattern.
THERAPIST: That's right! The more you wash, the more likely you are to wash again. This is why treatment is going to involve you touching something smelly and *not* washing'

Treatment

Mrs. K. was asked to cut up an onion *without* washing her hands afterwards 'You must be crazy Doctor, no one would do that', was her first reaction. However, when she came to see how this could break her 'ingrained behaviour pattern' by allowing her to habituate (that is become less anxious) she agreed to try. Her anxiety after cutting the onion on the 9-point scale was 8 (maximal), but after about 45 minutes reduced to 5 in the first session.

After two more sessions along these lines she was able to cut up an onion with an anxiety score of 4 at the start and 1 (minimal) at the end of 45 minutes. She then remarked 'The more I can do something *without* carrying out a ritual the easier it becomes, I think I can see how this idea could be used to solve my difficulty hanging up my dresses'.

She herself proposed to hang up the dresses without shaking them first 'but I know I am going to find this will make me very anxious'. She was told that her own idea was a good one, and that indeed it would make her very anxious at first, but that the level of anxiety would decline as it had done with the first behavioural task. This was, in fact, the case. The minor rituals to do with household chores were all dealt with in a similar way, and with similar success. Her husband greeted me towards the end of her treatment 'I know she does not want me to be involved in her treatment, but I just had to tell you she is a changed woman, I have not seen her so well and happy for years'.

Such cases emphasise the role that the therapist has as a *guide* as described by Pierre Janet (1925), and how dramatic change can be brought about (see chapter 1).

At this point it worth comparing exposure methods used for obsessive-compulsive disorders with those used for phobic disorders. Modelling is used in both cases and careful judgement of how fast to proceed is equally important. It is crucial in both cases to guide the patient on to the next step rather than using domination or cajoling.

The case of Mrs. K. is similar to a phobic disorder in that avoidance of contamination can be seen as similar to avoidance of the phobic situation by running away from it. Possibly self-monitoring and self regulation play a greater part in the treatment of obsessive-compulsive disorder. The therapist has to decide for each patient what a reasonable amount of time to spend on everyday activities such as washing hands before meals, taking a bath or getting dressed in the morning. In this way the therapist acts as a standard measure for the patient to decide what is normal behaviour. Another difference from treatment of phobic disorders is that they are usually more time consuming and intensive treatment often requires admission to hospital, as in the next case illustration.

Treatment of severe avoidance rituals and compulsive handwashing

Mrs. H. was severely disabled by not being able to touch her children, her husband or anything belonging to them. There was no clear-cut obsessional idea linked to her rituals although she thought they might have begun after her first child was born 13 years ago, and the ideas she then had about keeping the environment 'sterile'. She completely avoided dustbins and rubbish bins, and anything that had been in any way in contact with these objects. She had made the most amazing adaptations to her rituals: for instance she could do all the housework wearing plastic bags over her hands, and made her husband deal with the rubbish bins and clean the toilets. She avoided all lavatories except her own and had learned to hold herself several inches above the lavatory seat when using it. Just before admission to hospital she had begun to defaecate in a plastic bag which she would then bury in the garden.

In addition Mrs. H. could not go anywhere that involved proximity to or contact with water, particularly rain water or stagnant water. Short walks near to home that crossed bridges or went anywhere near stretches of water were avoided, greatly limiting her social and domestic life. She could not touch her children or her husband because they might have been in contact with a 'contaminated' object. The patient and her husband felt unhappy about the fact that they could no longer have physical contact and sexual intercourse was impossible. She could not touch her husband's pyjamas because they had been in contact with the bathroom floor. For similar reasons she could not touch her children, or any clothing or object that belonged to them.

Treatment

Three main goals were agreed:

1 To sit on a toilet seat and use it in the normal manner.
2 To touch her husband and his clothing in a more normal manner.
3 To touch her children and their clothing in a more normal manner.

The patient agreed that these were important and achievable goals worth striving for. However, in the first session there was difficulty finding a task that she could do, and she stated 'It's all too horrible, I can't do anything'. Nevertheless, she did eventually agree to try to touch her feet after walking on the bathroom floor. She was asked to rate herself on a 9-point rating scale, where 0 signified no anxiety and 8 meant she was extremely anxious. She rated herself 8 at the start of the session. By the end of the hour long session she rated herself 2. She also agreed to touch her shoes after walking on the bathroom floor, and her anxiety score was 8 at the start but 4 at the end.

Despite the success of the first session, the final goals seemed far away. The patient said ' You will never get me to use a public lavatory', and we could not persuade her to do so at this point. It was decided to incorporate imagery techniques to achieve the goal. The patient was asked to imagine she was sitting on a public lavatory seat whilst actually sitting on her own one at her home. Her anxiety at the start was 8, and had hardly reduced at all at the end of the session. Further sessions were carried out along these lines by a female nurse-therapist, and after four more sessions the patient agreed to use a public lavatory on the condition that the nurse checked it first.

By the eighth session it was decided to switch the focus to her inability to touch her husband. This was achieved by asking her to bring in a number of items belonging to him, and this she could do by using plastic bags to avoid ' contamination ' . These items, rated in order of the degree of worry they caused her were as follows: (1) shirt, (2) socks, (3) pyjamas, (4) shoes, (5) underwear. The therapist removed the shirt from the plastic bag, placed it on the table in front of the patient and said:

'I would like you to touch the shirt in the way that I am doing.' With this encouragement the patient did gingerly touch the shirt collar for which she was heavily praised. She was asked to hold her hand on the shirt a little longer and in this way gradually became able to handle the shirt with minimal anxiety.

In the next two sessions she learned to handle the remaining items of her husband's clothing, and could do so with an anxiety rating of 2 or less. For session 11 she brought items that belonged to her children, and these provided the focus for therapy along the same lines. She had not actually been able to touch her children for two years, but at this point felt able to go home and attempt this. At the start of session 12, with understandable emotion, she reported that she could not only touch her children but had given them a big hug. The patient and her husband were delighted with her success. At the last session she was given tasks to prevent avoidance developing, for example never to avoid public lavatories in future, to pick up and handle her husband's clothing at every opportunity, and to cuddle her children as much as possible.

Treatment of obsessive checking rituals

This next case illustrates how a trainee in psychiatry learnt to treat a patient with severe checking rituals. The patient, Mrs S., was a 55-year-old widow whose life was totally disabled by rituals. The trainee obtained the following history: Over the last six months, following the death of the patient's husband, checking rituals had started to take over her life. The main problem was an inability to trust her own eyes or believe in her own judgement. She could not leave the room without having to check all the angles of the room, and everything had to be in its correct place and look symmetrical, for example flowers in a vase all had to face the same direction. When she did the washing, she had to complete many checking rituals at least six times before she could start the machine. She had to put the plug in, switch the machine on, put the powder in the dispenser, shut the dispenser and then check again to ensure that the clothes were in the machine, and then again make sure the program was on the right number. Before going on to the next step she repeated the checking procedure six times. Before switching on the machine she felt very agitated, could not trust herself, and wanted to start all over again. She also said to herself 'Please God let it be right this time'.

The patient described her rituals as being like a nightmare and admitted to wasting more than half her day in these activities. Another time-consuming ritual was the compulsion to place the phone in a certain exact position, then to dust it, then to go upstairs and look down to see if the phone looked as if it was still at the correct angle. She then repeated this process going up and down stairs several times.

The trainee was then asked to try to uncover *feelings* the patient associated with the rituals and the following list was developed:

1   She feels angry with herself.
2   She asks God to help her get it right.
3   She promises God that if he helps her she won't do it again and this is the last time she will carry out the ritual.
4   She feels the rituals are silly and this leads her back to item 1 (feeling angry with herself).

During the next supervision session, the trainee discussed the relevance of the grief reaction in precipitating rituals, but it was decided that the patient had now come to terms with the loss of her husband, and it was not necessary to pursue grief work further.

In a typical session the trainee organised the rituals into a list of increasing severity (a hierarchy), and was given the task of discussing three specific points with the patient:

1   Arrange a meeting with the patient and patient's daughter together, so that the latter could learn to be a co-therapist.

2   Go through the obsessive-compulsive checklist with the patient.
     (See chapter 2 and Appendix 2.)
3   To discuss the use of modelling with the patient, e.g. the therapist
     disarranged her own telephone on her hospital desk, and encour-
     aged the patient to go home and do the same.

Following this, the trainee visited the patient's home and supervised
the patient disarranging her phone, and also asked her to remove things
from the refrigerator, and replace them in a disorderly manner.

Overall the trainee had nine sessions with the patient, whose anxiety
and obsessive scores on all measures improved. The patient was able to
go out of the house and lead a normal life free from rituals. The trainee
had the impression that the first three sessions were the most crucial and
the most helpful, and was impressed both by the importance of using a
relative (the daughter) as co-therapist, and the value of modelling in
treating a difficult ritual.

Another very difficult case describes how the therapist managed to get
treatment started despite a seemingly impossible problem: the patient
refused to speak about the symptoms!

The patient who could not reveal the symptoms

The first thing Mr. T. said was 'If I have to say the words I shall leave the
room and never come back'.

It was decided to ask him if he could *write down* the words, which he
agreed to do and dutifully brought the list to the next session. He called
this the list of 'unmentionables':

1   gas
2   gas-meter
3   gasman
4   tuberculosis
5   oil
6   methylated spirit

The therapist was now allowed to take the usual psychiatric history.
Mr. T was aged 25 years and divorced. He was a very successful
journalist. His problem using the above words started at age 20 after a
traumatic sexual relationship that he said was too painful to relate. He
then revealed that he had had five years of psychoanalytic therapy in
which many emotional problems were explored *but* had insisted that the
psychoanalyst never use any 'unmentionables'. He said that a traumatic
relationship had occurred with a woman who he subsequently discovered
had tuberculosis, and it transpired that the other items were variously
connected, for example he feared this person had tuberculosis, and the
woman had a boyfriend who was a gasman. Oil and methylated spirits had
associations with gas.

The symptoms interfered greatly with his life, for instance if he heard one of the words spoken on the radio, then he had to take all the clothes he was wearing at the time to the dry-cleaners, and carry out prolonged washing rituals that took most of the day to complete. In his job as a journalist he had to visit various places, but avoided doing so if he thought he might see a gas-meter. When walking in the street he always crossed over to avoid walking past a gas showroom, or an advertisement for a gas or an oil product.

Treatment had started when he had made the initial 'unmentionables' list. The problem now was to enable the patient to hear the words without carrying out rituals afterwards. He eventually agreed that the therapist could say the least troublesome word on the list *on condition* that the therapist allowed him to wear what he called 'battledress', by which he meant an old suit of clothes that he would not worry about getting 'contaminated'. With encouragement, he gradually allowed more difficult words to be spoken, and eventually the whole list. He no longer had to change clothes or carry out washing rituals.

Homework treatment tasks were set where he played a tape-recording of sentences made specially for him, containing as many 'forbidden' words as possible. He played this tape each evening, without washing afterwards.

In subsequent sessions he visited a gas showroom and brought leaflets describing gas appliances to the session to read out loud. A further homework task was to buy some oil for his car, and to put this in the engine. On the first occasion he did admit that he made the purchase from a self-service store! Later on he did go into an ordinary shop and ask for some oil. After this he gradually overcame all avoidance symptoms, and was able to work normally as well as lead an active social life.

The next case illustrates another variety of a compulsive ritual:

Treatment of hoarding involving the whole family

Mrs. L. felt compelled to hoard bills, household rubbish, and newspapers. As a result she had 300 newspapers on a sideboard and one room of the house was completely filled with rubbish. Washing her hands or clothing took at least four times longer than the average person. In the year prior to referral, her rituals had seriously increased, sleep was reduced, her sexual and marital relationships deteriorated, and her eldest son began to show abnormal behaviour.

The two main target problems were: (1) shopping without checking money or shopping list and (2) disposing of rubbish without checking contents. These targets were rated 6 and 0 by the patient on a 0- to 8-point scale, where 8 indicated maximum pathology. The first obsession occupied one to two hours each day and the second about one hour each day.

Involvement of the patient's family

Because her husband had been involved a conjoint interview was arranged. Mr. L. agreed to cooperate in preventing several of his wife's rituals. The marital relationship presented further problems: Mrs. L. constantly belittled her husband, and he teased his wife that his job was insecure. This served to increase her checking rituals. In early marital interviews the couple's attention was drawn to this, and they both made contracts to change their behaviour, using behavioural exchange therapy (as described in chapter 8).

Treatment of the checking rituals was carried out from hospital. Mrs. L. was taken by the therapist for shopping expeditions and not allowed to use a shopping list. The amount in her purse was altered so that she could not re-check it. At first she took a great deal of time choosing each purchase, and was very reluctant to let the therapist prevent her checking the change. Gradually she was able to purchase items with less hesitancy, and to adopt a more relaxed attitude to receiving change. Before her discharge from hospital the patient went home with the therapist, and further prevention of checking rituals was carried out in her car and at home. After Mrs L. had driven the car, the therapist instructed her to stop and leave the car without checking, and in the knowledge that the therapist might alter some of the switches. Mrs L.'s need to check the car rapidly diminished. The same applied to her difficulties with letter writing; she was asked to write several letters without checking spelling and punctuation, and to post these at once. Treatment continued after discharge with out-patient sessions, a home visit, and four additional conjoint marital interviews. During conjoint interviews the couple spoke more civilly to one another but there still remained problems at home. Husband and wife disagreed about the times they should go to bed and the arrangements for going out one evening a week. This was also treated with behavioural exchange marital therapy.

Despite these complications and the initial gloomy prognosis the patient made remarkable improvement and was able to throw away all the accumulated bills, newspapers and rubbish *after* she had overcome her need to check. By discharge she had improved to the point where she made only one check of car switches, dials on the stove, and the back door. The couple spoke more positively to one another and made decisions more democratically. At discharge the target problems were rated as 1 and 2 respectively, and neither obsession occupied more than five minutes per day.

This case shows how target problems can be decided despite the confusion at first sight. Obsessional patients often present a range of symptomatology and the therapist may be puzzled about where to begin. As in this case, the aim is to commence with a simple item 'not checking the shopping list' until this was mastered, then a more difficult item was tackled, until gradually fewer symptoms were present. The husband's involvement was crucial in this case before progress could be made.

Treatment of obsessive ruminations

This chapter began with a warning that the treatment of pure obsessions was difficult. This is because most patients have idiosyncratic emotional reactions associated with the rumination, and also because good clinical trials are difficult to conduct in this rare condition. These studies are reviewed by Salkovskis & Warwick (1988). Despite the complexities of obsessional ruminations, most of the associated emotional reactions fall into three categories:

1   The patient has a feeling of horror, disgust, or dislike.
2   The patient feels pleasure in a perverse way.
3   The patient feels insecurity and doubt.

Category 1 is analogous to washing and cleaning rituals, as in both cases there is an attempt to avoid something; in the case of rituals the washing serves to prevent contamination, in the case of horror-type ruminations the patient avoids thinking about the subject for prolonged periods, and the brief periods he does ruminate are not long enough for habituation to occur.

In this category the aim of therapy is to allow habituation to occur by persuading the patient to think the thoughts for prolonged periods as intensively as possible. This treatment is called **satiation therapy** and is analogous to exposure. The difficulty in producing this prolonged exposure has led to the development of new techniques called **habituation treatment** to prolong the exposure period.

Categories 2 and 3 are analogous to checking rituals in that their continued indulgence is reassuring, and so they become self-reinforcing. The patient finds it difficult to stop the checking rituals despite the realisation of their senselessness, and difficult to stop doubting-thoughts, which can be construed as cognitive checking (checking in the mind) in a similar manner. In these categories the aim of therapy is often to interrupt the thoughts by an external stimulus (such as a sudden noise), in such a way that the patient develops internal control over unwanted intrusive thoughts. This treatment is called thought-stopping. Recently, research has also examined ways of increasing exposure to the anxiety-increasing stimuli which result in this type of rumination, and satiation therapy is an attempt to achieve this.

Case illustrating satiation

Bill is a 20-year-old man with a rumination about the size of his nose. He cannot stop thinking about how disgustingly ugly his nose is, and this thought greatly upsets him. The thoughts interfere with his life and prevent him carrying out his studies at university. They also interfere with his social life and prevent him developing a relationship with a girlfriend. The last time he attempted an examination he could not write a word because thoughts about his nose kept intruding into his consciousness.

Treatment began by asking him to imagine that as he sat in the examination hall his nose grew to enormous proportions. He was then encouraged to let his imagination run riot and to speak aloud in an exaggerated way the worst possible consequences, with the therapist providing encouragement to keep going. Bill's words provide a good illustration of the technique:

I'm sitting there biting the end of my pencil trying to think how to answer the first question when the shadow of my nose starts to fall on the paper. I then find it has grown so big I can't see the paper at all. The other candidates turn round to look at me and I feel very foolish and embarrassed. The invigilator comes up to my desk and says 'You will have to leave we can't have freaks like you sitting this examination'. When I try to leave the weight of my nose makes it difficult to lift up my head. It has grown so large now I can hardly squeeze it through the exit. Once outside I give up all hope of walking home because of the weight of my nose, and hail a taxi. The taxi driver refuses to take me because I look so revolting. I'm left standing in the street while people jeer at me. Eventually the police are called but they can't get me into the back of the van as my nose is so large. They have to improvise a kind of trolley to put my nose on as I'm marched along the street. I end my days in a kind of side show for freaks . . .

This monologue was built up over three sessions and the patient then recorded it on a portable tape recorder, which he played to himself daily for three weeks. At the end of this time, habituation had occurred, and he was no longer preoccupied with thoughts of his nose to the same extent.

Case illustrating thought-stopping

A 27-year-old man could not stop worrying about whether or not he had performed small actions correctly. For 10 years he had worried about such things as turning off taps or the car ignition. He hardly ever went back to check these things but simply ruminated about whether or not he had performed them correctly. The symptoms had gradually worsened over the years so that he was currently unable to give anything his full attention, he could not concentrate on the job in hand, because of the thoughts of trivial actions and so his performance at work deteriorated.

Treatment

This consisted of 15 sessions each lasting 45 minutes, given three times weekly. The patient was asked to construct a list of his obsessions to use in treatment, starting with those that worried him the least.

Relaxation formed the first part of each session, the main aim of this being to enable the patient to concentrate on the subsequent cognitive task. When he was relaxed he was asked to imagine performing one of the actions that bothered him, for example turning off taps. When he had turned off the imaginary taps he was asked to ruminate about it for 15 to 45 seconds. A sharp noise was then made by the therapist clapping his hands and the patient was told to shout 'Stop!' simultaneously with the noise. It was explained that when he said 'Stop' the thought was supposed to go from his mind, which was, in fact, always the case. This was practised with further items in the list of ruminations. Eventually the patient merely said 'Stop' to himself sub-vocally and the thought went. He then practised the technique outside the clinic at a regular time each day.

This patient became very competent at thought-stopping, and was able to control the ruminations in the real-life situation. He described how going to work one day he had an obsessional thought about his umbrella falling off the rack, instead of worrying about it the whole journey, he relaxed in his seat and stopped the thought.

The part played by relaxation is unclear, but in general relaxation alone does not help obsessional symptoms. Relaxation possibly helps to focus the mind on the cognitive task of thought-stopping. Another ingredient of the technique is the sudden loud noise, which interrupts the rumination. As an alternative to the therapist clapping his hands, the patient could snap an elastic band on his wrist, or use any other mild aversive stimulus such as gripping a plastic hair curler that has sharp protrusions.

A further refinement of thought-stopping uses a small portable tape-recorder with headphones. The patient carries this around with a recording of a thought-stopping session, that can be turned on at an appropriate time. Some patients report that this is particularly helpful as the stimulus to stop the ruminations is experienced in a very intense way.

Case history demonstrating the use of habituation therapy with a personal stereo

Cecil, a 42-year-old unmarried ex-schoolteacher, had a 15 year history of distressing obsessional ruminations which occupied 10–12 hours a day and had led to his early retirement from work. Whenever he saw anyone he would have the thought. 'I would like to have sex with him/her'. This thought was repugnant to him as he was a devout 'born again' Christian who did not agree with extramarital sex and the idea of homosexuality, paedophilia and incest which his thoughts implied were abhorrent to him.

In order to reduce his anxiety, he had developed the habit of repeating the Lord's prayer and following this by saying 'Jesus, forgive me' seven times. If he was interrupted from doing this by any sound or movement in his environment, he would have to repeat it until performed perfectly. This problem had led him to seek the life of a recluse and he had even stopped attending church. He had contemplated suicide to rid himself of the problem but felt this was an even greater sin.

Initially, treatment took the form of graduated prolonged exposure to situations he avoided. However, he only made limited progress as he could not stop himself automatically starting his 'praying ritual' which helped to maintain his anxiety. It was decided that he needed to experience prolonged exposure to his anxiety-provoking thoughts without ritualising. This was achieved by getting him to record the thoughts (viz. 'I want to have sex with her. I want to have sex with him') onto a continuous loop tape in his own voice. The audiotape used was the type used for telephone answer machines. After recording this, Cecil was asked to play this to himself via a personal stereo with headphones for at least one hour, three to four times a day while in the company of other people, for example when on the bus.

Cecil found this so aversive initially that he had difficulty in complying. The therapist, therefore, advised him to start with the volume turned down low, and to increase the volume as he became more confident. This procedure worked extremely well and within two weeks of starting to use the tape, Cecil reported that he had little anxiety and was able to go out at other times. Despite having the thought, he no longer carried out the ritual. After two months he was able to return to work as a 'supply' teacher. At six month post-treatment follow-up, he reported that he had a girlfriend, was planning to marry, and he laughed at the thoughts which he now considered to be 'stupid'.

This technique using a continuous loop tape is only newly developed. Although its usefulness has been reported in case studies, at the time of writing it is still the subject of a controlled trial. However, in the experience of the authors, it has had a dramatic effect in several cases. Two issues appear to be of particular importance. Firstly, the tape should be recorded in the *patient's own voice* and secondly it should be played through the headphones of a *personal stereo*. The effect of both of these seem to make it virtually impossible for the patient to ignore the sound of the recording or to ritualise at the same time.

Summary

- Obsessive-compulsive disorder resembles phobic disorder but there are some important differences.
- Obsessional rituals serve to reduce anxiety, but this anxiety reduction is short lived, and then the ritual has to be repeated.
- Patients often have an anxiety-provoking obsessional thought, which is then followed by an anxiety reducing 'cognitive ritual'.
- The basis of therapy for obsessive-compulsive disorder is exposure to the anxiety producing stimuli, with prevention of avoidance.
- Common rituals are handwashing and checking.

- Involvement of the family in the ritual activity is not uncommon, and implies that treatment must involve the family.
- In patients with obsessional thoughts but no rituals, so called 'pure ruminators', recognised treatment approaches are 'satiation therapy ' which is analogous to exposure therapy, and 'thought stopping' which is analogous to response prevention.
- A further refinement of thought-stopping and satiation therapy involves the use of a personal tape recorder.

5   *Self-exposure*

The previous chapters have demonstrated the use of therapist aided exposure in the treatment of phobic and obsessive compulsive disorders. However, as well as performing exposure tasks with the therapists, each of the case histories also illustrated the importance of the patients continuing to practice exposure exercises on their own between sessions, and after completion of the course of treatment.

In the years 1960-70 exposure techniques often carried implicit instructions to patients that it would be therapeutic for them to practice going out into the feared situation in between actual therapy sessions. In retrospect, this variable may have explained the apparent effectiveness of weak exposure techniques like systematic desensitisation. It is impossible to prove this now as the variable of **self-exposure** was not controlled for in this early work (e.g. Gelder, Marks & Wolff, 1967). When later work showed imaginal exposure was also effective (Johnston *et al.*, 1976), the role of self-exposure was also considered. More recently, such 'homework' tasks have been shown to be vital for successful treatment (McDonald *et al.*, 1978).

The efficacy of this form of self treatment led to the development of self-help treatment manuals and packages. Recently, the efficacy of self-exposure has been demonstrated with a mixed group of phobic patients (Ghosh *et al.*, 1988) and also with patients with obsessive-compulsive disorder (Marks *et al.*, 1988). The case of Julie demonstrates how dramatically self-exposure can work.

Case history of Julie – the 'miracle' cure

Julie, a 45-year-old divorcee with three teenage children, presented with a 10 year history of fear of going far from home alone. Her problems had started at the time that her youngest child had been severely ill following a road traffic accident, and she had nursed him at home for several months. Since that time she had felt anxious when travelling away from home either on foot or by public transport. She had coped for years by doing shopping and making other journeys only when she was accompanied by one of her family. The reason for seeking help was her realisation that her family was now older, and that she would not be able to depend on one of them always being there.

A full history was taken and behavioural assessment was performed as described in previous chapters. After discussing the nature of anxiety, and the rationale for exposure, a number of treatment goals were agreed with her. Finally, some treatment targets for the week were agreed and she was asked to record her success in performing these as well as her anxiety level before, during and after the exposure practice. It was suggested that she might find the self-help manual *Living with Fear* (Marks, 1978) helpful to read.

A follow-up appointment had been made for Julie for the following week to discuss her progress and future goals. However, Julie was unable to keep this appointment as her youngest son unexpectedly won a prize at school and her appointment coincided with the presentation ceremony. She telephoned the hospital to rearrange this appointment but due to a bureaucratic error did not receive another appointment until four weeks later.

At her second appointment, Julie was extremely cheerful and full of self-confidence. She reported that during the first week, she had ventured out from home alone on foot, and had experienced a gradual reduction in her anxiety as she continued to practice. During the second week she had been pleased with her son's achievements at school and decided that she would like to buy him a new watch as a surprise. To be able to buy the watch which he wanted, she needed to travel into the centre of London alone. She, therefore, tried to buy the book *Living with Fear* to give her more guidance but had found that the only bookshop which had it in stock was five miles from her home. On an impulse she caught the bus to the booksellers, and to her surprise, found that although her anxiety was high, it was tolerable and it did reduce the longer she remained on the bus. Spurred on by her success, she continued to practise bus journeys and began to shop in increasingly busy areas. The day prior to her appointment, she had travelled by bus and underground train to London and had bought her son his new watch. Although she realised that she would still need to continue her exposure exercises to consolidate her gains, she felt optimistic about her abilities to continue.

The therapist praised Julie enthusiastically for her success. The need for continued exposure was reiterated to her, and arrangements were made to see her for follow-up to ensure her gains were maintained. The success of such self exposure methods, with their obvious advantage of increased cost effectiveness, may lead some readers to wonder if there is any need to train mental health care workers in the behavioural treatment of phobic and obsessive compulsive disorders at all. However, the reality is often more complicated than just giving a patient a book to read, and there are several reasons why firsthand experience of exposure is needed by the therapist. Firstly, whereas some patients seem to be able to read a

treatment manual and apply it to themselves without any further intervention, a substantial number cannot, without the additional motivatio-
nal factor of having to regularly report their progress to a therapist. In
addition the therapist is not only required to understand and be familiar
with the contents of the self-help manual, but may also need to explain
the exposure principle in alternative language, troubleshoot specific
problems, and be aware of potential pitfalls and problems. The case of
Tony demonstrates this role of the therapist.

Case history of a young man with an inability to understand self-help manuals

Tony was a 19-year-old single man who worked as a labourer at a building
site. He had always been a reserved and shy person, but since leaving
school at the age of 16 years he had been unable to eat or drink in public
for fear that he might spill the food or drink on his clothes and 'make a
fool' of himself. His problem had caused him to become an avid reader of
self-help manuals about anxiety. Tony's reading ability was limited but he
had managed to plough through some of the good and not so good books
about his problem, but he still felt he did not know what to do to
overcome his problem.

   After taking the history, the therapist started to explain the principle of
gradually facing up to feared situations. However, Tony had a blank
expression and obvious difficulty in grasping the concept. The therapist
drew a number of graphs and pictures to try and explain more clearly but
to no avail. Eventually the therapist asked:

What would you tell your work-mate if he had an accident in his truck and was
scared to drive again?

Tony replied:

I'd tell him he must face it and get back in the truck.

   The rest of the session was spent agreeing situations with Tony in which
he could gradually *face* his feared situation, and a simple written record
was given to him to fill in his successes.

   Thereafter, Tony continued to make progress with his self-exposure
programme until in session five, he reported that he had been more
frightened, and had started avoiding some situations again. Careful
enquiry revealed that as Tony had become more confident, he had started
going to the pub in the evenings for a drink. Following a particularly
heavy drinking night, he had felt jittery and anxious when due to have his
lunch on the building site with his friends, and since then had avoided
eating or drinking with them. Alcohol can be a form of avoidance during
exposure, and even modest amounts can make people feel more 'jittery'
once the immediate effects have worn off. This was explained to Tony,

who agreed to restart his programme sticking to low alcohol and alcohol-free beer.

Tony progressed well with his self-exposure programme and at one-year post-treatment follow-up had started dating a girl, who worked as a waitress in a fast-food restaurant and was spending many of his evenings sitting drinking coffee and waiting for her to finish work before they went out.

Despite Tony's experience, there are some excellent self-help manuals for phobic and obsessive compulsive disorders (e.g. Marks, 1978; Mathews, Gelder & Johnston, 1981). However, some patients do not seem to fit neatly into the categories described and need a more individually tailored programme. Jane had a problem which, despite her reading several self-help books, she could not decide how she should start treating herself and wondered if she might have a unique problem.

Treatment of a young woman presenting with dysphagia

Her GP referral letter described Jane's problems as:

This patient has difficulty in swallowing solid food, and investigations including a barium swallow and endoscopy showed no abnormality. Could this be a hysterical condition such as globus hystericus?

Jane, a pleasant and intelligent 24-year-old staff nurse on a coronary care unit, arrived at the clinic apologised profusely for 'wasting time with such a silly problem'.

She had always been a rather shy and retiring person but had gained confidence in herself after starting her nursing training. The previous year she had moved to her present job, which she enjoyed. However, shortly after changing jobs, she had separated from a long-standing boyfriend. The break up of this relationship was unexpected and she felt miserable for several weeks after. At this time, she was eating her lunch in the hospital canteen and experienced difficulty in swallowing. Her friends had commented on the fact that she had left her food. Following this episode she had difficulty in swallowing solid food and described a sensation of it sticking in her throat. This problem was worse when she was in company and reduced when she was alone. Consequently, she had stopped eating in the staff canteen and refused all dinner or lunch invitations.

The therapist then explained how the initial symptoms of difficulty in swallowing had been precipitated by her distress following the end of a love affair, and was now maintained as a symptom of anxiety. Avoidance of eating in public increased her anxiety about these situations, and made it more likely that the symptom would recur. The rationale of exposure treatment was explained, and Jane decided on some treatment targets for the following week.

Jane completed a self exposure programme to the feared situation over the next 6 weeks. To begin with she had chosen to eat semi-solid foods like minced beef in the company of close friends and had sequentially moved up the hierarchy to eating solid food in a restaurant. The therapist's role had therefore been to disentangle what had seemed to Jane to be an inexplicable problem.

Unlike Jane, some patients are either too anxious or too incapacitated to even start to attempt self exposure without some modelling and therapist aided sessions. Samantha was a young woman with obsessive-compulsive disorder who was too anxious to initially attempt self-exposure.

Self-exposure treatment of obsessive-compulsive disorder requiring initial therapist-aided exposure

Samantha was an 18-year-old girl who had worked as a nanny but was, at the time of referral living with her mother and younger sister. She presented with a 10-month history of fear of contamination by urine and faeces which had led to her losing her job. The problem had started three months after the death of her father and had seemed to be precipitated by her watching a television programme about the risks of hepatitis to health care workers. Following this programme she had become nervous that she might contract and spread hepatitis to other people. Although she recognised that her fear was exaggerated, she felt unable to prevent herself from taking elaborate precautions to prevent 'contamination'. These precautions included washing her hands at least 40 times a day; bathing for three hours nightly; avoiding touching door handles or other objects, which had been handled by people unknown to her or only touching these items using paper tissues; any clothes which had been worn by her were placed in a plastic bag immediately following removal and were not allowed to come into contact with 'clean' clothes, and if she felt she was not entirely 'clean' and free of 'contamination', she would be unable to sleep in her bed at night (a designated 'clean' area) but would sleep on the sofa.

After the assessment of the extent of the problems, and educating both Samantha and her mother about the rationale of treatment, Samantha agreed to start an exposure programme at home with her mother acting as co-therapist.

The next week, Samantha and her mother returned to the clinic. Both looked disappointed and apologetically reported that they had been unable to make any progress. The targets for the week had been that, with the help of her mother, she was to touch her 'dirty' clothes and then systematically 'contaminate' all her clean clothes and to sleep every night in her bed even if she did not feel perfectly clean. However, when Samantha had attempted her first exposure programme, she became more anxious than she had anticipated, and had wept profusely and begged her mother to stop the exposure and to help her to wash and check that her clothes were clean again. Initially, her mother took a firm line and reminded Samantha of all that the therapist had told them. After a while, the sight of her daughter crying uncontrollably and shaking with fear was too much for her and she relented and complied with Samantha's demands.

As these items of exposure had been rated by Samantha as the easiest ones to start with, it was difficult to think of ways in which the programme could be made less anxiety provoking. The therapist, therefore arranged to visit Samantha's home to help her with this exposure exercise.

When the therapist arrived at the house, Samantha was already extremely anxious and tearful. The therapist sat down with her and her mother, repeated the rationale for treatment, and reassured Samantha about the success of exposure treatment and that her anxiety would reduce if she faced up to her fear. Eventually, Samantha appeared more settled and agreed to take the risk of touching her external clothing and then the outside of her wardrobe and chest of drawers where her clean clothes were kept. During this exposure, she was noticeably tremulous and tearful but managed to continue. She was praised by the therapist for her success. Once she had finished this contamination exercise, she agreed to try and touch all her clean clothes. She systematically handled all her clean clothes and was surprised to find that her anxiety *did* reduce as she continued, although she remained concerned that her fear might escalate after the therapist left. Before completing the session, Samantha volunteered to 'contaminate' the bed clothes of her clean bed. Once she had done this, the therapist again praised her, and arranged to telephone her the next day to monitor her progress, and to encourage her to continue practising the exposure twice daily.

Following this therapist-aided exposure session, Samantha progressed extremely well. She reported that once she had 'taken the plunge' and found that her anxiety did eventually reduce, it was possible for her to continue and increase the difficulty of the exposure tasks. Over the next six weeks she practised exposing herself to situations of increasing difficulty, including public lavatories, initially with a total ban on hand-washing and bathing and eventually reintroducing 'normal' washing activities. Returning to work as a nanny was her final target which she achieved two months after her therapist-aided session.

Conclusions

Finally, if a therapist is to give advice and help a patient to plan an exposure programme, it is imperative that he or she not only understands the theoretical background to the techniques, but also should understand and have experience of the practicalities of the treatment and how to cope with difficulties, as well as to fully appreciate the distress and discomfort which patients may experience during exposure. These are best *learnt by the therapist* accompanying a patient during exposure. The case of Samantha in this chapter demonstrated how lending a sympathetic ear to the patient's fears and encouragement to try out exposure can be needed. In chapter 3, the case history of Adrian's experience at the airport also illustrated how profound the symptoms of anxiety can be with many patients, and how the therapist's observation that Adrian's hyperventilation was adding to his distress could then be remedied.

Summary

· Self-exposure is as successful as therapist-aided exposure for many patients, and is so effective in the great majority that clinician-accompanied exposure is redundant.
· Even if self-exposure techniques are used, the therapist needs to understand fully the rationale and practicalities of this treatment.
· Some patients are too anxious for self-exposure alone.

6 Reduction of undesirable behaviour

The previous chapters have concentrated on altering maladaptive fear responses using the exposure principle. However, other maladaptive habits or behaviours may develop in response to stimuli unrelated to fear and in these cases alternative strategies may be needed. In these cases the therapist has the option of:

1   Eliminating the behaviour using **aversive therapy** (only indicated when the behaviour is life-threatening or a severe public nuisance), e.g. **covert sensitisation**.
2   Modifying the stimulus resulting in the response, e.g. **orgasmic reconditioning**.
3   Modifying the response to the stimulus, e.g. **stimulus control techniques**
4   Replacing the problem behaviour with alternative adaptive responses (**competing response practice**), e.g. **habit reversal**.
5   Reducing the desirability of the problem behaviour e.g. **mass practice**; **response cost**.

These five categories are not mutually exclusive and any therapist who tries to eliminate a particular behaviour without helping the patient to develop alternative strategies is doomed to failure. The case of Giles illustrates how a particular technique can be used in a treatment plan.

Covert sensitisation, sexual and social skills training used to treat sexual deviancy

Giles was a 25-year-old man who was referred to the Clinic by the probation service. He had recently finished a prison sentence for his repeated offenses of indecent exposure to young women in the local park. Despite his custodial sentence, his probation officer had reason to believe that Giles had re-offended since his release.

The full psychiatric history was difficult to obtain from Giles who appeared a shy and diffident man who avoided eye contact and answered questions in brief, non-discursive replies. He was the only child of elderly parents and had led an isolated life. His school years had been unhappy as, although an average scholar, he had been bullied by the other children and had eventually refused to go to school developing symptoms of school phobia and refusal. Referral to the child psychiatric services had not resolved this problem and he had been taught in a tutorial group with other 'delicate' children. Thereafter, having finished his education without gaining any formal qualifications, he had obtained a job as a warehouseman, preferring his solitary life. He had never made any friends at school or in his employment and had never had a girlfriend or any sexual relationship.

The history of his sexual development was that he had reached puberty at 13–14 years of age. No formal sex education had ever been given to him and most of his knowledge he had picked up from the television, tabloid press and 'girlie' magazines. He masturbated once a week to heterosexual fantasies.

The history of his public genital exposure began at the age of 19 years. A sexually explicit magazine had included a story about a man who exposed himself to women. It had implied that this was very erotic to many of the women, who were then overtaken by passion and made love to the man in the park. Giles had been enthralled by this story and began to emulate this man.

He would wait until he was alone at home and would then play some erotic music and look at a 'girlie' magazine. After this he left the house and went to the park. At this time he would be extremely sexually aroused, and would be fantasising about making love to his favourite 'porn' star.

When at the park, he would wait behind a secluded clump of trees near to a footpath. His ideal victim was a woman of 16–30 years with blonde hair and alone, although he would sometimes expose himself to a group of women. Once he had seen his target, he would come out from the trees and stand on the footpath exposing his genitals. If the woman appeared shocked and ran away, Giles would find this arousing as he believed that she would think about the episode and find it erotic. On occasions, however, women had laughed at him or shouted abuse, which he found deeply distressing, and which resulted in his not returning to the park for several months. If he had received a preferable response, he would return to the trees and masturbate. His masturbatory fantasies for the next few weeks would then focus on this episode until he would return to the park again four to six weeks later.

During the first session the behavioural analysis revealed that Giles would need four components in treatment i.e.:

Sex education.
Reduction in deviant urges.
Increase in socially acceptable sexual activity.
Improvement in general social skills.

The deviant behaviour, therefore, was the first item which needed tackling, in order to avoid Giles being arrested again and so being prevented from completing his treatment programme.

During the second session a full description of the arousing situation was obtained. This included full descriptions of the surroundings in which Giles performed his activities, as well as descriptions of his thoughts, emotions and fantasies. A similarly detailed description of three aversive scenes were also obtained from him. These were:

1   I am exposing my genitals to a woman and she starts to laugh. Her face creases with delight and mirth. She is pointing at my genitals and laughing. As she gets her breath back she says 'Look at that tiddler, call yourself a man, I have seen babies that are better equipped.' She then calls to three friends who arrive on the path. They all look at my genitals and laugh uproariously. They make comments to each other like 'It must be a caterpillar' and 'I would not show us that, Love, you may lose it.' I turn and run but can still hear their laughter and taunts in the background.

2   I am exposing my genitals and I suddenly feel the arm of a man on my shoulder. I turn round to see this six-foot man with a skinhead haircut. He has tattoos on both arms and looks very angry. 'What are you doing, that's my girl', he says, 'I'm going to have to teach you a lesson.' He punches me in the face, I feel the pain but immediately I feel another punch in the stomach and then in the face again. My head aches, my nose is broken, I'm on the floor, he's kicked me in the genitals. All the time he's cursing and shouting at me. I'm laying on the ground as a helpless bundle, so weak I cannot move. He takes out a long, thin knife and picks up my penis, 'Now for the best bit', he says . . .

Giles had great difficulty thinking of a third aversive scene connected with his deviant behaviour, and so the third scene was non-specifically aversive.

3   I feel dreadfully sick. My stomach is churning and my hands and forehead feel cold and clammy. I'm having difficulty in standing up straight. My legs are weak. I collapse and fall into a large vat of liquid. I go under and realise that it has a revolting pungent smell. The liquid is semi-solid and sticky. I realise that I have fallen into a huge vat of vomit . . .

The therapist then recorded, using a 0 to 8 scale, how arousing the sexually deviant scene was to Giles and how aversive the three unpleasant scenes were. It was, however, easy for the therapist to observe that Giles looked animated and excited when describing the arousing scene and pale, tremulous and anxious when describing the aversive scenes. Indeed, if this had not been the case, the therapist would have had reason to try and identify alternative fantasies.

Giles was then asked to sit in a comfortable chair in a relaxed position. He was asked to imagine the arousing scene in detail and to verbally repeat and describe his fantasy. The therapist prompted Giles with details if he appeared to be flagging. Before reaching the end of the pleasurable fantasy, the therapist instructed Giles to switch to the first aversive scene and describe this in detail.

During the first session this pairing of pleasurable and aversive fantasies was done four times. Giles was then asked to do the same exercise himself at home three times a day. To aid his imagination, he was asked to write down a 'script' for all the scenes describing the fantasy in as much detail as he had done in the session.

In the application of covert sensitisation, it is important to establish at least three aversive scenes. This is because the patient will be frequently exposed to the aversive scene and habituation of the anxiety would render the aversive scene useless. Therefore the therapist needs to prescribe different aversive scenes, and to frequently check that the aversiveness ratings of the scenes remain high.

Over the next six weeks, the therapist saw Giles for weekly sessions during which the fantasy pairings were repeated at least six times in every session and were continued by Giles between sessions. The aversive scene was gradually introduced earlier and earlier in the 'pleasurable' scene.

At the sixth session, Giles reported that he no longer found the arousing scene pleasurable and had extreme difficulty in inducing this fantasy without experiencing symptoms of panic. It therefore appeared that the covert sensitisation had worked extremely well, particularly as Giles explained that he had tested this out by trying to walk to the park, but had felt so anxious that he had had to return home.

The next problem to be tackled was establishing appropriate sexual behaviour. During the previous six weeks, the therapist had asked Giles to read some basic educational books about sex, because all his prior sexual knowledge had been obtained from 'girlie' magazines and was thus inadequate and biased. These new books were discussed with Giles to ensure that he had understood the information. Appropriate sexual fantasies which were acceptable to him were then discussed. It transpired that although Giles had previously masturbated, he had always used the unusual technique of lying face down on the floor and rubbing his genitals against the carpet. This produced low levels of arousal which had been increased by his deviant fantasies. The therapist explained the technique of masturbation using manual stimulation, and Giles was asked to practise this at home while using *appropriate* fantasies.

While Giles was being instructed in sexual education and masturbation training, he was also attending a social skills group which used the techniques of rehearsal, modelling, feedback, role play and homework practice, as described in chapter 7.

Three months after the commencement of treatment, Giles reported that he had a girlfriend whom he had met at an evening class on car maintenance, which he had been encouraged to join by the social skills group. This later developed into a sexual relationship which was satisfactory to both of them. He had no deviant urges and fantasies any more, and reported that he was much happier and enjoying a social life.

In the case of Giles, it was clear that his antisocial sexual behaviour was causing a public nuisance which required immediate action to prevent him being arrested and given a further custodial sentence. In these cases, rapid treatment to suppress deviant sexual urges based on aversion therapy are justified. Even in this case, however, a successful treatment plan incorporated other elements to increase his general levels of social functioning. Not all cases of deviant sexual behaviour are so clear cut. If a patient has a sexual preference which worries him and is a cause of concern to his sexual partner, but is not in itself dangerous or causing a public nuisance, then less radical treatments may be used.

Orgasmic reconditioning is a technique frequently used in these cases which was originally described by Marquis (1970). In this treatment, the patient is asked to masturbate regularly to his troublesome deviant fantasies but, at the point of orgasmic inevitability, to switch to the desired, 'non-deviant' fantasy. As treatment progresses the non-deviant stimulus is introduced earlier and earlier in the arousal process, until masturbation is achieved without the deviant fantasy. Following this, further sexual or social skills training is usually needed to ensure that the arousal to non-deviant stimuli is maintained.

When dealing with troublesome sexual urges it is important to set realistic goals with the patient. Whereas a bisexual man who wishes to become exclusively heterosexual may be helped by appropriate orgasmic reconditioning and sexual skills training, it is not possible nor usually desirable to change the orientation of an exclusively homosexual individual. In this case, counselling to help him or her accept their sexual preference may be needed. Similarly, if a homosexual paedophile is referred for treatment, it would be unrealistic to set the goal of regular adult heterosexual contact, but adult homosexual orientation is more likely to be achievable.

The preceding case histories have all featured male patients. This is because sexual deviancy is rare in women, but other problem behaviours have a more equal sex distribution.

Treatment of obesity

Obesity is a common problem in the Western world and has been generally not amenable on a wide scale to medical, psychodynamic and the early behavioural approaches. The development of behavioural treatment packages in the 1960s were much more successful (e.g. Stuart, 1967). These packages consisted of four key elements:

1   Description of behaviour to be controlled. Patients are asked to keep daily diaries of amount of food, time and circumstances of eating.
2   Modification and control of the discriminatory stimuli governing eating. Patients are asked to limit their eating to one room, to use distinctive table settings and to make eating a 'pure' experience unaccompanied by other activities, e.g. reading, watching television, etc.

3   Development of techniques to control the act of eating, e.g.
    counting each mouthful of food and replacing utensils after each
    mouthful, always leaving some food on the plate at the end of a
    meal.
4   Prompt reinforcement of behaviours which delay or control eating.

Case illustration

Joyce was a 35-year-old housewife with two young children. She had been
overweight during her teens but had lost weight when she had started
work as a telephonist and had maintained a normal weight until the birth
of her eldest child 10 years earlier. After the birth she had stopped work.
She had gained two stones in weight during pregnancy but believed that
this would reduce with breast feeding. Her weight did not reduce and she
tried several strict dieting regimes during which she would lose a few
pounds and then binge and regain the weight. Her younger daughter was
born five years earlier and at the end of that pregnancy, she was five
stones above her ideal weight. Again she would diet for a few days with
good intentions, and then a minor crisis in the home or boredom would
lead her to break the diet. Once she had eaten a 'forbidden' food she
would feel a failure and eat anything that was readily accessible to try and
comfort herself. Joining a slimming group had not helped and she had
even been to a private slimming clinic to ask about surgical techniques.
    At the first session, the therapist performed a full behavioural assess-
ment of the problem, ascertaining that Joyce would eat well balanced
meals of normal size three times a day but that her 'binges' would occur at
other times. She would feel the urge to eat if she was miserable or bored.
The food chosen was whatever was readily available and had ranged from
a packet of biscuits, the childrens' Easter eggs or a pound box of
chocolates, bought as a present for a friend and eaten in frustration at a
bus stop when the bus failed to arrive on time. This eating was normally so
rapid that she hardly tasted the food and was generally performed with
her standing or walking. Following a 'binge' she would feel guilty, a
failure and disgusted with herself.
    Her husband was a supportive and loving man, but he had started
treating her weight loss attempts as a joke and told her that she would
always be 'big' and 'cuddly'.
    The therapist asked Joyce to eat normally over the next two weeks but
to note down in a diary every food that she consumed. As well as
recording the quantity and type of food she ate, she was asked to note the
time, place and circumstances as well as her mood before and after
eating. It was emphasised that she was not to diet, but to eat absolutely
normally.
    Joyce arrived at the second session looking very pleased with herself as
she had lost four pounds in weight by just monitoring her food intake. The

diary demonstrated that sadness and boredom were likely to result in 'binge' eating. Joyce was then instructed about some other measures she was to introduce. Her knowledge of nutrition was good due to her extensive reading about diet. She was asked not to diet, but to eat three well-balanced nutritious meals a day. At no time was she to starve herself or feel hungry. If she was hungry at other times she could eat a 'snack' and should keep nutritious 'snacks' like tomatoes and low fat yoghurts in her refrigerator at all times. The only restriction on her was that she should only eat in the dining room, sitting at the table and using a red place setting and serviette. Whenever practical, the food should be eaten with a knife and fork. While eating she was to concentrate on what she was doing, was not to read, listen to the radio or television. Between each mouthful, she was to place her utensils on the plate. Solid food should be chewed at least 15 times for each mouthful. She was only to eat enough to satisfy her hunger and should leave some food on her plate at the end of a meal or snack.

As well as controlling her general eating patterns, certain 'problem' situations were identified by Joyce and the therapist. Certain foods led to her eating in excess. Biscuits and sweets were a particular problem. Joyce agreed that the safest thing for her to do was not to buy them, even for the children. Instead, she would give them fruit as treats. If her mother gave sweets to the children, Joyce was to keep them in a large tin with a notice on it which read:

These are not for you, Joyce, they are for Graeme and Sophie. Stop, think and do something to occupy yourself!

Waiting for the bus to go to the shops was another difficult time as it was near a sweet shop and the boredom of waiting frequently led Joyce to buy sweets. She decided that the best way would be for her to walk to the shops which was only a few stops away and catch the bus back. At times when she felt miserable or bored in the house Joyce compiled a list of alternative pleasurable activities she could do. These included:

Having a bubble bath.
Washing and setting hair.
Manicuring nails.
Reading a chapter of a book.
Taking the dog for a walk in the park.
Riding my 'trim cycle' for 10 minutes.

A ban was put on her weighing herself, as weight loss is slow and prone to fluctuations, and Joyce had become disheartened in the past when she thought she was not proceeding fast enough.

It was important that Joyce should reward herself for sticking to her programme. She decided that she would save sufficient money from not buying sweets and chocolates for herself, and by walking to the shops to be able to buy herself a new lipstick and nail polish at the end of the week. Further suggestions for *rewards* at the end of subsequent weeks were also made.

At the end of the session, all of the rules of the programme as well as the lists of problems and strategies were written down and given to her. She was also asked to continue keeping her food diary, and to also note times of temptation and the strategies she had employed.

Over the following two months, Joyce was seen weekly to monitor her progress with the behavioural programme, to 'troubleshoot' any difficulties and to receive reinforcement and encouragement from the therapist. At the end of this time she had lost two stones in weight and had gained much confidence. It was therefore decided to reduce the visits to the clinic to monthly sessions.

Six months later, Joyce had reached her target weight having lost over five stones. As the regime had not involved any strict rules of dieting, it was relatively easy for her to gradually increase her food intake to maintain this weight, and not too revert to her old eating habits. Joyce was asked to gradually increase her portions of nutritious food until her weight (measured fortnightly) was stable. It was explained to her that this was the most difficult time of the programme, as research has shown that whereas many people can lose weight, most people regain weight again once they 'relax' their rules. For this reason, it was arranged that Joyce should visit the Clinic for the usual one-, three- and six-month follow-up and thereafter continue to attend every six months to help increase her incentive to keep her weight stable. In addition, Joyce had joined a slimming club in her area, and was keen to continue attending this as a further motivating factor to maintain weight loss.

Two years later, Joyce remained at her ideal weight. She was an animated and busy person who had recently retrained and returned to work. In addition she was an active member of a squash and tennis club. Both Joyce and her husband were delighted with her success, and she reported that her marriage and general health had greatly improved.

This case history demonstrates how addictive behaviour can be modified using a number of techniques which modify the stimulus, the response and the reinforcers of the response. Similar strategies can be used for other addictive behaviours including drug and alcohol abuse. The main difference between these problems and obesity is that frequently a total abstinence is the desired goal, whereas total avoidance of food is obviously not a reasonable goal for the obese patient.

Treatment of alcohol abuse where abstinence is advisable

Shug, a 55-year-old unemployed Glaswegian labourer, had a 40-year history of excessive drinking. This problem had resulted in the loss of numerous jobs, the separation of himself from his wife and children, and his social and financial deterioration. When referred to the clinic, he had already been detoxified from alcohol but, as this had been a frequent occurrence in recent years, he had attended to see if we could improve his situation in the longer term.

His physical health had been greatly affected by his drinking behaviour. His liver function tests were grossly abnormal, and he had a history of duodenal ulceration and haematemesis. Previous treatment had included referral to self-help groups, and a six-month attendance at an outpatient clinic for supportive psychotherapy.

Behavioural analysis of Shug's problem demonstrated that, although he had achieved abstinence in the past for several days and weeks, if he once took a drink he felt that he had lost control and would then continue to drink until he passed out or his money ran out. He would previously drink at any time of the night or day and whether he was alone or in company. Previous periods of abstinence had broken down when he had received his social security benefit, and had then seen friends going into a public house or off-licence.

Treatment commenced with the therapist discussing ways in which Shug could avoid some of the stimuli which precipitated a drinking bout, or to control his access to alcohol once he had started drinking. Plans were made with him to move into a hostel and to attend Alcoholics Anonymous, for example, to try to increase his social contacts with people who were abstemious. He also agreed to only carry a maximum of £5 at any time, changing his habits by collecting his benefit from a Post Office which was adjacent to a branch of his bank.

Shug, however, felt that these actions would be insufficient to maintain his motivation to remain alcohol free. He said that he felt he would need to be 'locked up' for six months if he were to be able to permanently stop drinking. It was therefore decided that he should be prescribed disulphiram (Antabuse) to help his will-power.

Disulphiram is an agent which, if alcohol is taken following its administration, causes vomiting or occasionally, more severe reactions (see *British National Formulary*, 1990, pages 201–2). It should only be prescribed in a hospital, specialised unit or by clinicians experienced in its use, because of these potential reactions. A test dose of alcohol following disulphiram is a useful test, and demonstration of the effects to the patient but should be performed in the controlled setting of the clinic.

Shug agreed to try disulphiram which was prescribed for him, and arrangements were made for him to be admitted to hospital for a day for a test dose of alcohol. The test dose of alcohol caused Shug to vomit profusely and to feel nauseous for six hours after its ingestion. Theoretically, this experience acted as an aversive stimulus which was paired with the previously pleasurable activity of drinking alcohol. Future temptation to drink alcohol reminded Shug of the likely consequences of drinking following disulphiram and increased his will power.

Although the pairing of the extremely aversive experience of nausea and vomiting with alcohol might be thought to be a sufficiently noxious experience to produce abhorrence of alcohol for ever, this is unfortunately, rarely the case. Whereas, many people have long-lasting aversions to certain foods if they have symptoms of gastroenteritis following their ingestion, the previously pleasurable associations of alcohol seem to impair such *one trial learning*.

Shug did not react by permanent avoidance of alcohol. Generally he was able to reduce his drinking, but at times of stress would stop the disulphiram for a few days and go on a drinking binge. These binges have occurred at a frequency of approximately three month intervals.

Four years after starting therapy, Shug has considerably reduced his drinking, but has not achieved the goal of abstinence. Although his drinking is sporadic it follows a 'binge and out of control' pattern. Attempts to introduce controlled drinking have failed. On the positive side, however, he is now working as a night watchman and has held this job for two years. His employers have been tolerant of his occasional absenteeism due to alcohol. The general physicians are less worried about his physical health but would still wish him to be alcohol-free.

Unlike Shug, in some problem drinkers moderation is required rather than abstinence and a controlled drinking programme based on similar lines to Joyce's programme, but substituting alcohol for food can be used. The teaching of controlled drinking is still thought by some to be controversial, although there is increasing evidence for its efficacy in selected cases. In some cases there are definite contra-indications: for instance the presence of organic damage due to alcoholism, as any amount of additional alcohol intake could worsen this damage. As this important area is outside the scope of this volume the interested reader is referred to Sobell & Sobell (1978).

Problem behaviours may also take the form of bad habits which have been learnt in response to a whole range of stimuli. Azrin & Nunn (1973) pioneered the treatment of habit reversal which has been used to treat a range of nervous habits including multiple and facial tics, nail biting and neurodermatitis. This treatment has four components:

Awareness training.
Competing response training.
Habit control motivation.
Generalisation training.

These four elements are illustrated in the case history of Sarah.

Treatment of facial tics using habit reversal

Sarah, an attractive and lively 24-year-old games mistress was referred to the clinic with a 14-year history of unsightly and embarrassing facial tics.

The onset had occurred at puberty, but was not related by Sarah to any particular life-event. Over the years she had received treatment with a variety of medication including haloperidol and the benzodiazepines, to no effect. She had also received individual psychodynamic psychotherapy which had not helped.

The tic could occur at any time but was more frequent if she was anxious or bored. Close observation of the movements revealed that it commenced with Sarah screwing up both eyes, followed by crinkling her nose, and then making a sharp downward movement of her chin opening her mouth.

The first thing that Sarah was asked to do was to record the frequency of her tics over a few days. This **awareness training** is useful, as many people with habit disorders are oblivious of some of the times when they perform the undesirable behaviour. Obviously, Sarah had a busy life and so the records were made as simple as possible for her to keep. She was asked to obtain a small notebook and to divide each page into columns each representing a one hour period. Every time she performed the tic, she was asked to place a mark in the appropriate column. Also she was to record her activity at each hourly interval e.g. lunch with colleagues, lacrosse lesson with Lower Sixth Form.

This diary was also useful as a baseline measure of Sarah's problem, and was maintained throughout treatment to monitor her progress. In addition, the therapist decided to use another assessment measure by recording an interview with Sarah on videotape for a 20-minute period. During this interview, the therapist asked a series of 'neutral' questions about her job and hobbies and some more emotive questions about the effect of the tic on her life. The mean number of tics per minute during the 'neutral' and 'emotive' discussion was then calculated and this procedure was repeated at the end of treatment with the therapist asking identical questions. The baseline measures showed that Sarah performed the tic an average of 300 times a day or approximately 0.5 tics per minute.

At the second session the principle of **competing response practice** was explained to Sarah. The therapist said:

> One of the problems with a long-standing habit is that you have built up and strengthened the muscles of your face which are involved in the tic at the expense of the opposing muscles. What I will be asking you to do is to perform some exercises to strengthen these opposing muscles.
>
> The start of every tic begins with you screwing up both your eyes. As soon as you feel that you are going to tic, I want you to raise your eyebrows, wrinkling your forehead. You may find this easier to do if you place your thumb and index finger of one hand under each of your eyebrows. I then want you to hold this position to the count of 20 or until the urge to tic passes, whichever is the longer time. At the same time as doing this I would like you to clench you teeth together very tightly and likewise to maintain this position.

Following this description, the therapist asked Sarah to practise the competing response in the session. The therapist then asked Sarah to list all the deleterious effects of having a tic and the advantages of being tic-free. She was asked to write this list down and to read it through whenever she felt bored or disheartened by the treatment (**habit control motivation**).

Finally, ways in which Sarah could incorporate the competing response movements into her everyday life without looking conspicuous were discussed. Sarah suggested that if she were outside, she could place her hand under her eyebrows as if shielding her eyes from the sun. If she was inside and sitting at a desk or table, she could use her hand under her eyebrows to support her head (**generalisation training**).

When Sarah was seen a week later for her third session, the frequency of tics had already reduced to less than 10 per cent of the baseline level. Difficulties were discussed with her at this session, and over the following two sessions.

Six weeks after her initial appointment, Sarah was discharged from active treatment. The frequency of tics was less than one per cent, which was acceptable to Sarah. This improvement was maintained at one-year post-treatment follow-up.

Although habit reversal is a very rapid and effective treatment for many patients with habit disorders, some patients fail to respond. Mass practice was a treatment devised by psychodynamic psychotherapists which can sometimes be used for patients in whom habit reversal has failed or is inappropriate.

Repetitive throat clearing treated by mass practice

George, a 56-year-old road sweeper had been treated for tuberculosis of the lung five years earlier. Since that time he had developed the habit of repeatedly clearing his throat despite having no phlegm to move. This habit occurred 60–80 times an hour and was causing some marital problems as it greatly irritated his wife.

Treatment with habit reversal had been unsuccessful as it was difficult to find an effective competing response for George to use.

The therapist then decided to use mass practice. George was first asked to find three half hour periods in the day when he could retire to his room alone and would not be heard by his family. He was then told that during these times he was to repeatedly clear his throat for the entire 30 minute period. At other times of the day, he was to try not to clear his throat but to 'save it up' to his next throat clearing session.

The week after this instruction was given to George, he returned with his wife to the clinic. He reported that he had complied with the instructions for the first three days but that since that time the thought of clearing his throat was so aversive to him that he had not been able to do it at all. His wife confirmed his improvement, and was delighted with it. George was asked to continue monitoring his throat clearing, and to reintroduce mass practice if the frequency increased to more than five times a day.

Summary

· Maladaptive habits or behaviours may develop in response to stimuli unrelated to fear, and in these cases a variety of strategies may be needed.

· Eliminating the behaviour using aversive stimuli is only indicated if the behaviour is life-threatening or a severe public nuisance e.g. covert sensitisation.

· The stimulus that produces an unwanted response can itself be modified, e.g. orgasmic reconditioning.

· The response to the stimulus can be modified, e.g. stimulus control techniques.

· The problem behaviour can be replaced with alternative adaptive responses, e.g. habit reversal.

· The desirability of the problem behaviour can be reduced, e.g. mass practice and response cost.

7   *Social skills training*

One definition of social skill is 'the ability to express both positive and negative feelings in the interpersonal context without suffering consequent loss of social reinforcement' (Bellack & Herson, 1979). This strictly *behavioural* definition ignores many of the complexities of social behaviour. One way forward is to emphasise that the socially inadequate person may fail in two main ways:

1   Social phobia: this is similar to other phobias and is dealt with in chapters 3 and 5.
2   Lack of skills acquisition, and this may be the result of a:

        lack of *social skill* per se
        lack of *assertiveness*
        lack of *impulse control*

Shepherd (1983) suggests that social competence may have three components:

1   The observed *behaviour* during a social interaction.
2   The *cognitive responses* a person makes in a social interaction, that is their subjective thoughts and feelings, and how competent they feel themselves to be.
3   The ability to sustain social *roles and relationships*, e.g. as a father, teacher, employer, colleague or friend.

Social skills training that naively focuses on behaviour alone, the so called 'eyebrow school' of social skills is generally inappropriate in the psychiatric setting, but might have a role in other settings such as management training, and in schools. In the psychiatric setting the multifactorial model is advocated.

The treatment approach in social skills training will vary depending on the clinical condition. It is based on the notion that the skills are learnt and therefore can be taught to those who do not have them. The techniques depend on research by social psychologists and others in the study of non-verbal behaviour, speech and conversation. One model suggests that people behave socially according to rules and that they monitor performance depending on continuous feedback from the environment (Argyle & Kendon, 1967).

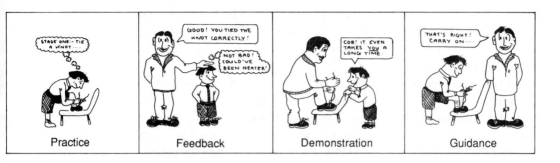

Fig. 7.1. The principals of skills acquisition.

The principles of skills acquisition include:

>Practice
>Feedback
>Demonstration
>Guidance

These principles are illustrated in Fig. 7.1.

Anyone who has ever taught a child to do up his shoe-laces knows the importance of *practice*. Most people also learn complex tasks best if the task is broken up into smaller components: first teach the child a simple stage in tying the knot rather than the whole thing all at once. Another factor in practice is whether to have a few long sessions or many short sessions: there is conflicting evidence here, spaced sessions being best for most learning tasks, but massed sessions have proved best in treating some phobias. For social skills it is probably best to have sessions long enough to complete a reasonable amount (about 45 minutes), and sessions spaced far enough apart to allow homework tasks to be completed (about once a week, or once every 2 weeks). Another important factor in teaching social skills is *feedback*. In the case of teaching a child to do up shoe-laces, the feedback is both *intrinsic* and *extrinsic*, and the same is true of social skills learning. Intrinsic feedback comes from the child himself: he can see if he is getting anywhere with the knot, and if prevented from doing so either by distraction, or visual handicap, progress would be thwarted. Extrinsic feedback comes from the parent saying whether the knot is being tied correctly or otherwise. In social skills training the therapist praises the good aspects of the performance, and it has been suggested that positive feedback, that is praise, is more effective than criticism. It should also be as detailed, specific and highly focused as possible. Feedback should be in non-technical language and should focus on behaviour which the patient should be able to change. The use of audiotapes or videotapes can assist in providing feedback, if the equipment is available.

Demonstration as in showing how to tie a shoe-lace, is crucial in social skills training. The person who gives the demonstration, known as the *model*, should give a *coping* rather than a *masterful* performance, showing that although he has difficulties ('Oh dear, I have not done so well this time') he is effective in the end ('Worth the effort now I have finally succeeded'). Once more videotapes can be effective, and greatly save on therapist time.

Guidance in psychological therapy has a long history (see chapter 1) and in social skills training is a method of ensuring the patient performs the correct movements in the initial stages. Although guidance is very useful in the early stages the therapist must guard against too much guidance *after* the initial stages of therapy, as it is possible that the patient will become dependent on the guide and too afraid to make his own mistakes.

Plan of therapy

Firstly the main problems to be dealt with in social skills training are drawn up. Then the best techniques for dealing with the problems are decided. Guidance and demonstration are usually used early on, followed by practice and feedback.

This will be illustrated by a case example in a young man unsuccessful in interpersonal relations, partly because he was phobic in these situation, but also because he had not acquired the appropriate social skills.

Lack of social skills: a case illustration

Jeffrey was hiding beneath a newspaper in the waiting room, and when called for his appointment did not look up but kept his eyes firmly fixed on the floor. During the interview he did not look at the therapist, and his voice was barely audible. In muted tones he described how he had always been shy even at school, since when he had gone to university but shyness had prevented his joining in with social activities. Then he had trained as a librarian and enjoyed his job, except when this brought him into contact with the public. His shyness in this situation had been noticed and was threatening to hold up his promotion. He always ate sandwiches alone to avoid dining with colleagues, and his social life was very poor as he feared going out into social situations and so had become a complete recluse. His main spare-time activities were watching television alone or playing chess with a computer. The most fearful situation for Jeffrey was talking to a young woman when he would become lost for words and feared blushing.

Assessment

Jeffrey had a poor opinion of himself and thought that he would fail in certain situations even before he tried. This expectation of failure had become a self-fulfilling prophesy, and that was why he never met young women. He now totally avoided the feared situation, and had become a recluse. This made him think even more badly of himself, and so the vicious spiral continued.

Treatment

This followed four stages:

1 A description of new behaviour that was to be learnt.
2 Learning of new behaviours through the use of guidance and demonstration.
3 Practice of the new behaviour with feedback.
4 Transfer of new behaviour to the natural environment.

Description of new behaviour to be learnt

This was achieved by asking Jeffrey in what ways he thought his behaviour ought to be changed:

THERAPIST: Tell me Jeffrey what would you like to do, that you find too difficult or painful at the moment?
JEFFREY: I suppose I ought to be able to look you in the face.
Then I'd like to be able to talk to people without blushing.
I would like to be able to eat in front of other people, especially at work.
And finally he admitted in a whisper:
It would be great if I could chat to women like other blokes do.

These four statements were taken as goals to be aimed for in the next phase of treatment.

Learning new behaviour through guidance and demonstration

The problem of gaze aversion was dealt with by guidance and demonstration. Firstly a co-therapist and therapist demonstrated how they looked at each other during a conversation, and Jeffrey was asked to watch this. When the therapist asked him to copy the behaviour, however he reverted to his habitual gaze aversion. He was then given direct training in looking the therapist in the face:

THERAPIST: I am going to look *you* in the face and I want you to stare directly back at me, no matter how hard this is, do not look away.

After having stared at each other for two minutes, the therapist asked him how he felt and he said, 'most uncomfortable, I wish the earth would open and swallow me up, I feel hot and red, and very embarrassed.'

Despite these feelings, it was possible to encourage Jeffrey to carry out brief periods of mutual gazing, while the other looked away. The time spent looking was slowly increased, until he could tolerate it for five seconds.

Next the time spent looking was gradually increased, first of all with the therapist speaking while he listened, and finally he spoke whilst the therapist listened. At the end of six sessions along these lines he no longer felt hot and uncomfortable.

This deliberate staring was a method used to encourage direct exposure to the feared situation. Staring itself is not usually socially appropriate, and some time was then spent discussing with the patient the *rules of eye contact*. That is, brief contact with the eyes is made on first meeting someone, it is useful to make brief eye contact again when making a point, but direct eye contact is broken and intermittent during normal conversation. It is also usual to make brief eye contact on parting.

After repeated practice he gradually become less worried about looking the therapist in the face for prolonged periods, and he was given homework tasks to look at other people such as his landlady while engaging them in conversation, obeying the rules of eye contact.

Practice of the new behaviour with feedback

We next made a videotape of an interview between Jeffrey and a friendly female medical student. The student was a socially skilled attractive young woman who asked Jeffrey all about his work in the library. When the videotape was played back he was seen to make good eye-contact and was praised for this. In general it is best to begin by emphasising *positive* behaviour, before going on to negative criticism. On the negative side it was immediately clear that his conversational skills were poor, he never initiated conversation, and he spoke in a soft, barely audible voice.

It was then suggested to Jeffrey that in the next videotaped session he should prepare some questions to ask the student, for example, how she chose to go to medical school and what she liked about it.

When he attempted this last task he became completely inaudible on the videotape feedback, and attention was now focused on his problem with voice production. Before this he was given *positive* feedback for the things he was doing well, e.g. his posture was better. He was then encouraged to practise after each had been modelled:

> The use of an expressive tone, and the therapist demonstrated how this could be done first.
> Speak fluently, again this was demonstrated.
> Speak faster, also demonstrated.
> Use powerful speech, also demonstrated.

To this end he carried a card into the next session on which with these four instructions were written. He soon began to use a more expressive tone, but had to guard against developing a high pitched voice. Fluency likewise increased with practice, especially when he had formulated his thoughts in advance, something he was learning to do. As his confidence increased he was able to increase his speed of speech from an initially painfully slow pace. His speech also became more powerful with practice and exposure to the situation, and he was given a few rules to help this, e.g. avoid the use of prefatory remarks such as 'I think,' 'I guess,' 'I mean,' 'sort of,' 'you know' and to avoid expressing *uncertainty* by making statements that sound like questions.

Whenever he used a good expressive tone, spoke fluently, spoke faster or more powerfully, the achievement was pointed out and he was praised.

Transfer of the new behaviour to the natural environment

Jeffrey had done well so far and had exceeded his own expectations, but still worried about his performance in the real-life situation. However, he now agreed to meet his colleagues in the work cafeteria and coped with eating in front of them with little difficulty, possibly because they all happened to be men: his greatest difficulty remained talking to young women.

There were very few situations where he came into contact with young women, and his social skills deficit was partially responsible for this self-perpetuating situation. One possibility, however, was on his weekly visit to the launderette.

JEFFREY: I dread having to speak to someone so I usually take a book along. I know I would not be able to say anything to a young woman.
THERAPIST: Leave the book behind and initiate a planned conversation with a young woman, which we will have previously rehearsed

This was along the lines of 'Could you show me how to work this machine?' This turned out to be very successful, as the young woman then talked to him in a non-threatening way about the neighbourhood and he was able to practise his new found voice production and conversational skills.

Later on some sessions were spent with the aim of improving his lifestyle, and he realised that playing chess with computers was not helpful. He joined a social club for University graduates and in this way was able to meet young women in a non-threatening environment where his new skills soon generalised, his social roles expanded, and he continued to improve to follow up at one year.

Variations on the basic training

In some cases therapy is not as straightforward as just described and if difficulties are encountered, more complicated techniques can be used:

Role play and role reversal

This is where the patient plays the role of someone he fears encountering, e.g. in the case above Jeffrey could have pretended to be a young woman, and the therapist could have taken the role of Jeffrey himself. In this way the therapist would have acted as a competent model so that the patient could be exposed to a useful learning situation. In the next stage the patient plays himself again and the therapist plays the young woman.

Use of an ear-microphone

This is a device for the patient to receive prompting from the therapist who watches the session through a one way screen. It could have been used in the case above if the patient had been totally lost for words, as is the case with some patients.

Use of a script

Once again, for the patient who becomes speechless in certain situations a script can be useful. The patient himself can be encouraged to write the script as a homework exercise and it can be discussed and edited with the aid of the therapist. Reading from the script in practice sessions is gradually faded out, so that it is eventually not necessary in practice sessions before carrying out real-life practice.

Use of a self-help book

In our experience many patients with social anxiety have read some self-help books with little success. This could be because some of these books are not that helpful for patients with serious disorders. On the other hand some patients with specific problems, making conversation can be helped by reading *Conversationally Speaking* by Alan Garner (1980), and using material from that book as a 'script' for practice sessions.

Lack of assertiveness: an example of assertiveness training

Jo was a 35-year-old woman who described herself as lacking in self-confidence since birth. She had been 'shy' as a child and remembered being teased at school. The presenting complaint was that she felt she could never stand up for herself. When asked for a current example she described how people took advantage of her at the office where she worked as a supervisor in a computer factory. She had her own office but other workers would often come in to talk to her and smoke a cigarette. There was a no smoking policy at work, and Jo herself was a non-smoker who found cigarette smoke very irritating. She said that she could never tell her workmates to stop smoking in her office in case she caused offence. She also felt that she was taken advantage of in other ways, for instance if her boss gave her extra work she could never refuse, although she knew that she already took on more than the other supervisors, and she would have preferred to spend her spare time in other ways.

Plan of treatment

The assumption in this case was that the patient had acquired the habit of giving in to people from an early age. The thought of standing up for herself made her anxiety increase, so she took the line of least resistance in a situation of conflict and became compliant. However, her compliance then made her angry and frustrated with herself, and she often became depressed as a result.

The aim of therapy was to establish some realistic targets for her to learn to increase self-confidence.

Treatment

In discussion, it became clear that she needed to confront her workmates over the smoking issue but she had no idea of how to tackle them. The therapist therefore worked out a way of doing this and role played the patient using the following dialogue:

> I think you ought to know that I strongly disapprove of smoking at work. It is nothing against you personally, but cigarette smoke irritates me very much, and there is a policy about smoking in our factory. As a supervisor here I have been letting you get away with it for too long already, but from now onwards I would be grateful if you would go to the smokers' room when you want to light up a cigarette.

The patient then played herself in this assertive role, and the therapist played the role of the workmate, who acquiesces about going off to the smokers' room. Role play along similar lines was used to tackle the problem of the boss taking advantage of her.

In similar cases there are a number of standard situations where patients can be asked to practise assertive behaviour:

> Go to an expensive car sales shop and ask for a test drive.
> Go to a chemist's shop, order a large supply of condoms in the hearing of other customers, and ask for a discount for buying a large supply.
> Enter a private art gallery with a view to buying a picture and then changing one's mind.

Despite the seemingly frivolous nature of these examples they have all been used to good effect in actual cases. An important warning here is that patients are never advised to do anything that might be potentially damaging to them or their careers. Clearly, reciprocal negotiations between patient and therapist are crucial and prior agreement about the task to be attempted must be clear: a patient would never be given the task of telling the boss that he was self-opinionated and superannuated, even if this was true.

Lack of impulse control: an example of anger management

Bill was a 20-year-old who wanted help because of outbursts of anger and sudden flare-ups of temper. He was perfectly friendly at the assessment interview, but described situations when he felt a sudden impulse to hit anyone who happened to be around at the time. He was asked to describe the last time this had happened:

PATIENT: I was talking to this friend of mine and things started to get rather heated, it all got out of hand and I hit him.
THERAPIST: Can you tell me exactly what you where talking about.
PATIENT: It was about motorbikes, I remember now, he said something about my bike I can't repeat in polite company. The thing was he was running down my machine if you see what I mean, and I'm very sensitive about that.
THERAPIST: What happened at that point?
PATIENT: I just saw red. I don't think I stopped to think at all. The next thing I remember was him lying on the floor all covered in blood. I was very worried then. He was just lying there and my next thought was that I might have killed him. Then the ambulance came.

Treatment plan

In carrying out the standard assessment it was clear that Bill was often violent after he had had a few drinks. It was also clear that certain sensitive subjects made him likely to hit out at the person he was talking to. He himself thought that he hit before he thought. The situations were those in which he considered someone to be critical of him. He was near to tears with remorse when he talked about the incident afterwards with the therapist.

The goal was to try to interrupt the behavioural chain whereby disinhibition of behaviour (probably due to alcohol) lead to sudden flare up of anger, which led to a violent action.

Treatment

Bill was not dependent on alcohol, but after some discussion was able to accept the association between drinking and disinhibited behaviour and agreed to stop drinking for at least a trial period.

He himself wanted to do more than this and was motivated by the incident he described above, because he thought he might have killed someone at the time, although he realised afterwards that he had not. He was asked to think of what might have happened if his worst fears proved to be well founded, and to describe these thoughts, 'I would feel very guilty, I don't think I am basically a violent person. I am shocked by my own actions.'

THERAPIST: What do you think should happen to you if you did injure someone in an accident?
PATIENT: I should have to go to Court and face the consequences.
THERAPIST: What would the worst consequences be?

PATIENT: I imagine going to prison, my case would be reported in the newspapers, I would be so ashamed when my family and friends saw that.

The next four sessions were spent in going over in detail exactly what happens when he is prone to become angry. At the point where he noticed the anger *just starting,* he was asked to visualise the worst consequences as described above, and to elaborate on these to make them realistic and aversive at the same time. After four more sessions he reported a success in the real life situation where he had been teased by on of his friends, but managed to summon up the aversive imagery, and not to give way to the impulse to hit his friend. He reported a return to social drinking without relapse of symptoms six months latter.

This case was successful partially due to the good motivation, and the ability to use visual imagery to good effect. The technique has similarities to that described in the case of exhibitionism, which also deals with the reduction of undesirable behaviour (chapter 6).

Personality Disorder

In contrast to the above case, in personality disorder the problem is not usually one of overcoming anxiety, low self esteem or lack of confidence. Here the difficulty is that a whole range of antisocial and often destructive behaviours have become reinforcing for the patient, and the problem is how to reverse this.

Clara, aged 25 years, had been admitted to hospital after setting fire to her flat. Prior to this she had been admitted on numerous other occasions for taking overdoses of tablets. After the last overdose she had been told by her psychiatrist that she would *not* be readmitted following an overdose, because this was reinforcing her maladaptive behaviour. Clearly this therapeutic strategy had failed, and had resulted in an even more dangerous action (setting fire to her flat) which had the additional effect of rendering her homeless.

She gave a history of long standing difficulties maintaining relationships which had reached a climax two years earlier after the breakup of her marriage. Because of her disordered behaviour her husband was given custody of her two children, and since then her behaviour had deteriorated further. She had taken to travelling on public transport without paying the fare. When asked to pay the fare she would remove her clothing. This usually had the effect of the police being called, and she would then tell them about her sad life and previous psychiatric history, which would result in readmission to a psychiatric hospital. When in hospital she had a range of disordered behaviour: nurses described her as 'childish and attention seeking', for instance she would go up to other patients and tip over their cup of tea. She would often shout abuse, and take off her clothing in the middle of the day room. At one time she urinated beside her bed, although staff were convinced that she was perfectly capable of getting to and using the lavatory.

Assessment

This was initially very difficult as Clara had learnt how to mimic the symptoms of other patients on the ward and at various times gave convincing demonstrations of *manic* or at times *schizophrenic* behaviour. However, the staff consensus was that she was imitating these illnesses to gain attention. Hospital had become a safe, rewarding place where she found kind staff willing to listen to her problems. In the outside world she was expected to fend for herself, and she had no real friends or family in this country that she could turn to for support. Deviant behaviour, e.g. taking off her clothes in public, was something she used to gain attention and emphasize her status as 'patient'. As the caring professionals found her increasingly tiresome and difficult to control, and increasingly negative in their reactions with her, she responded by becoming even *more* difficult. Thus the vicious spiral of behaviour continued.

Treatment

A behavioural programme was constructed with the objective of halting this vicious spiral, and giving Clara the opportunity to learn more appropriate behaviour.
The following behaviours were measured:

1   Shouting and screaming.
2   Being physically aggressive.
3   Taking off clothing in inappropriate places.
4   Urinating on floor.

The first three behaviours occurred three or four times each day, but the fourth only once in the week when these base line measures were taken.

In order to change the reinforcement contingencies for these behaviours, Clara was put in a room by herself whenever they occurred, a procedure known as **timeout**. This is a procedure which can vary greatly in the manner in which it is carried out, and is similar to methods used in dealing with the chronic patient (chapter 10). In the treatment of this case it involved removal from positive reinforcement for periods of one to four minutes, that is the patient had to remain in a separate room with no contact with staff or other patients during this time.
Timeout was used for a total of 13 hours in week 1, and for a total of seven hours in week 2; a dramatic reduction in deviant behaviour.

Next, a system of *points* and *rewards* was used to reinforce positive behaviour. This was established by finding out things that Clara *liked* to do. She liked having certain members of staff to talk to, and so a staff member was nominated to spend 30 minutes each day with her if she had earned an agreed number of points for acceptable behaviour. She also liked letter writing and going out for walks, and so these behaviours were also earned by acquiring points. She gained an average of 9 points per day during week 1, which is equivalent to 4 hours of acceptable behaviour. The number of points gained increased by 60 per cent in the second week, and the period in timeout dropped by 50 per cent. This was a clinically significant improvement in behaviour, but it was noted only with hindsight as the staff implementing the programme at the time were not aware of this.

As the timeout was less needed it was gradually phased out, and the behaviours rewarded by points included activities outside the hospital. On the fourth week she went on a shopping trip with a member of staff, and later on was allowed to visit a public house. She chose to accumulate points for favourite activities, and it was noted by week 6 that there was a dramatic improvement in her appearance and level of interests. In this way it was possible to eliminate all the deviant social behaviours, and arrange for positive behaviour to be reinforced in the community.

The point system was then gradually phased out, and the dramatic clinical improvement continued. She no longer indulged in destructive behaviour, no longer took her clothes off in public and in general was socially acceptable to those around her. In cases such as this, it has been noted that relapse may occur when time out, and the point system of rewards are stopped. This was not so in this case, possibly because the treatment was brought in at a particularly dramatic moment, or because it allowed the patient to 'start life again' with a new set of people where it was no longer necessary to use such attention seeking behaviour.

The range of applications of social skills training

Smooth social functioning is at the centre of much human activity, and the range of applications of social skills training is wide, as illustrated in Fig. 7.2.

Social skills problems are a component in the many psychiatric illnesses, but central in the conditions described above – social anxiety, and conditions where skills acquisition is poor. They are also of considerable importance in the treatment of depression and chronic schizophrenia. The depressed person may be unable to show behaviour that is positively reinforced by others, will generally lack assertiveness, and show a low level of activity. The management of these problems in general is described in chapter 12, but may often include a social skills training component, as described here.

In chronic schizophrenia the lack of social skills may be a function of the disorder, and the effect of institutionalisation, whereby the individual has never had the chance to learn appropriate social skills. The emphasis

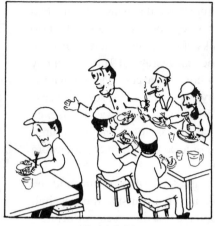

Social phobia

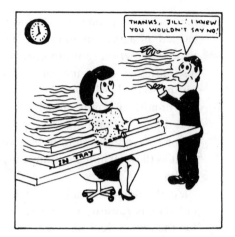

Lack of assertion

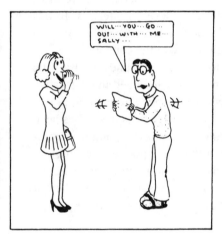

Lack of skills

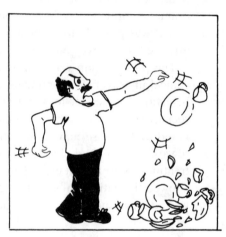

Impulse disorder

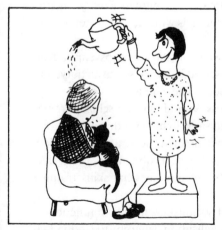

Antisocial personality

Fig. 7.2. The range of social skills applications.

here is on the *deficit* aspect of the disorder, although many techniques are similar, e.g. practice, rehearsal and praise are used in both conditions. The treatment techniques for schizophrenia are described in the chapter dealing with the chronic patient (chapter 10).

Individual versus group treatment

Many of the techniques used in treating individuals can be applied in a group setting. There are similar advantages and disadvantages to that of group treatment for agoraphobia, described in chapter 3. The groups would need to be *homogenous*, that is all neurotic disorder patients, or all personality disorder patients, as well as all having the same level of skill at the start of the treatment programme. There is a potential saving in therapist time if patients are treated in groups, but the treatment goals must reflect the needs of the whole group, and in practice it may take some time to put such a group together. A specific advantage of the group is that individual members may role play for one another and can provide feedback and reinforcement for each other. However, the progress of the group may be likened to that of a convoy at sea: it can only go as fast as its slowest member.

Group training has certain advantages in teaching social skills training to therapists, where one therapist has considerable experience and the other is new to the techniques. Therapists also report that carrying out treatment in this way is more enjoyable. Research has not yet shown whether group methods have enough to recommend them to be widely applied.

Summary

- Social skills training applies both to social phobia, and lack of social skills acquisition.
- The principles of skills acquisition include: practice, feedback, demonstration and guidance.
- Lack of assertiveness requires specific techniques such as **role play** and homework practice, directed at the low level of assertiveness.
- Lack of impulse control can be dealt with by anger management: a package of techniques directed at training recognition of early cues that trigger the impulse.
- In certain varieties of antisocial personality, there is scope for operant training techniques (**operant conditioning**) aimed at teaching socially acceptable behaviour using methods similar to those used with chronic patients.
- Due to the wide range of applicability of social skills training methods, the techniques may be referred to throughout the book, but are brought together in this chapter.

8 *Behavioural marital therapy*

'All happy families are alike but an unhappy family is unhappy after its own fashion' was noted by Tolstoy, at the start of his novel *Anna Karenina* (1878). This accurate observation makes it difficult to describe the complexities of marital difficulties using only a few cases. Nevertheless, in this chapter we shall focus on the *behavioural* aspects of therapy, fully realising that there are many other models of marital therapy. In reviewing this field Jacobson & Gurman (1986) describe four 'major models' and six 'emerging models'. One of the major models is behavioural, and described by Jacobson as the 'social learning-cognitive (SLC) model'. The SLC model includes:

1 Behavioural exchanges.
2 Communication and problem-solving training.
3 Other techniques, including sex therapy.

Behavioural Exchanges

The application of social learning theory to marital therapy is attributed to the pioneering work of Stuart (1980) who recognised the power of the patterns of mutual reinforcement that married couples set up. He also suggested that the way to enable one partner to change behaviour is for each to make an initial behaviour change, and the way to initiate the change was to reward each partner for carrying out the behaviour change that had been suggested by their partner (Stuart, 1969). An illustration of the problem is shown in Fig. 8.1.

Following the work of Stuart, Azrin *et al.* (1973) described a similar technique they labelled 'reciprocity counselling'. There is clearly a plethora of terms with similar meaning; so for the sake of simplicity we shall call all such interventions **behavioural exchange therapy.**

Case illustration

Mary and Ron were a couple in their 30s with a three-year-old child. Ron worked in a firm of accountants and was successful at his high powered job. Mary had given up her secretarial job to look after their child, and was happy to do this. The problem this couple had was one of 'constant

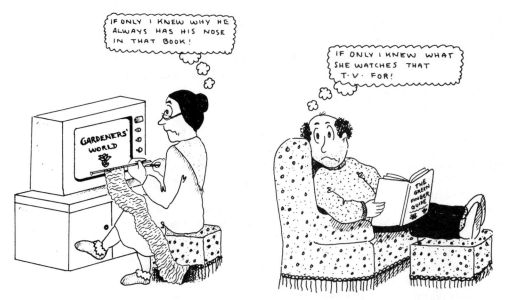

Fig. 8.1. One partner has to initiate change.

rows', and each of them gave the following account when seen together and asked to say what they considered to be was the main difficulty:

MARY (who spoke first): He is becoming impossible to live with . . . I never know what time he will be home at night . . . and in what condition . . . I mean how much he will have been drinking.

RON: Well, there is not a lot I can say in my defence. I know I have behaved badly. The thing is it's the job. Most of the people I work with go out for a few drinks, one thing leads to another, and before long I just forget all about coming home.

THERAPIST (to Mary): You have said Ron is impossible to live with, and then you specified his coming home late, and then his drinking too much. Is that the main thing that you would like to change about Ron?

MARY: Not just that. I could cope with that. When I found out about the womanising, that was the last straw.

THERAPIST (to Ron): It would be helpful if you told us here all about that.

RON: Again, I can't defend myself, except to say it was one of those things all the lads did at the office. After a few drinks we would go on to a club, and one thing led to another. Mary would not have found out except that I had to tell her when I got a sexually transmitted disease. I don't blame her at all for being angry, about that. We have talked about it all, and Mary has been good enough to forgive me. But still we have constant rows.

THERAPIST (to Mary): *Constant* rows?'

MARY: No I would not say the rows are constant. They are only after he has been out for one of his evenings, and comes back late.

Assessment

The impression was one of negative feelings predominating in this relationship. Ron's behaviour led to Mary's anger, and this only served to make his behaviour worse. The therapist next asked each of them to tell the other the ways that each might change things that each most disliked in the other. Initially this met with some further hostility, Mary said 'he will talk to me as long as he is sober enough'.

This negative barb was pointed out: Mary wanted him to talk to her *and remain sober*. The therapy proceeded to enable each to point out truly positive ways to change.

Treatment

THERAPIST: Could we agree here over what is reasonable behaviour on Ron's part. Do you think, Mary, he should never come in late, and what time would you both think is late?

MARY: One evening a week I would agree to, and I need to know in advance which evening. Also he should never be so drunk that he behaves really badly, and absolutely no more sexual infidelity.

THERAPIST: Is this reasonable?

RON: She is absolutely reasonable about the sex. But, I do have to entertain clients in the evening, usually more than once a week. My job, and therefore our income depends on that . . .

THERAPIST: Can either of you think of a way round this problem.

MARY: There is no reason why he could not phone and tell me if he was going to be late. If he did this, I would accept that he could be late, up to twice a week.

THERAPIST: It looks as if you two have agreed on something, and I would like to summarise: Ron is allowed out late up to twice a week, *on condition* that:

1   Ron telephones home
2   Ron does not get drunk
3   Ron stops womanising.

At this point the therapist wrote down for the couple the agreement they had just made and asked them to sign it. It was pointed out that it had been valuable to spend time discussing the problem in this way. They were given the homework task of setting aside an agreed amount of time each day for discussion. They both agreed to spend one hour each evening in this way. Another homework task was for each to make a list of things they would like to change in their partner if they could, and they were to bring the lists to the next session.

At the next session these lists were read by the therapist, and it was decided to investigate further one of the items on Ron's list that seemed to be a complaint about Mary: 'Mary likes to go out with one of her girl friends, and this makes me angry.'

THERAPIST: (to Ron): I would like to know why you get angry about this?

RON : I know you are going to say it's not fair of me to expect to go out with my friends, and not to let Mary do the same! The point is that I can't help getting jealous. I imagine her and her friend getting picked up by a couple of men.

THERAPIST: What is the evidence that this happens?

RON: Well, they look so happy when they come home, and I know Mary is an attractive woman.

THERAPIST: Is this any proof?

RON: Not really, but I can't help getting that thought, even though it makes no sense.

THERAPIST: What do you think of all this Mary?

MARY: I think he is crazy to be jealous like that, and there are no grounds for it. He does say sometimes that the clothes I wear are too sexy, and he asks me to change them sometimes. I resent this, as I consider my dress to be most modest usually.

THERAPIST: It sounds as if Ron's insecurity about Mary going out does not have good justification. Can either of you think of a way to help?

MARY: I don't see why I should stop going out.

THERAPIST: That does not seem fair, I agree.

RON: If she gave me a big kiss before going out, I would find it much easier. Also if she did not wear the red dress.

THERAPIST: What do you think of that?

MARY: Sounds fine to me.

This dialogue illustrates how the therapist acts as an arbitrator to help a couple isolate a problem, and work towards a solution, which involves compromise on both sides. Once the behaviour (Mary going out) was identified, it had to then be *specified* what it was that Ron was worried about. Then it was necessary to stop Mary reacting in a *catastrophic* way (not going out at all) and mutually agreeing a compromise. The intervention can be described as *cognitive* because the meaning Ron ascribed to Mary's behaviour was just as important as the behaviour itself.

This session led to a discussion of adoption of roles within marriage and marital stereotypes. To continue this discussion at home they were asked to read a popular book entitled *Families and How to Survive Them* (Skynner & Cleese, 1983). We recommend this book with reservations, because it uses a mixture of techniques only some of which are behavioural. However, there is at present no other popular book on this topic that is better, and of particular value are the amusing illustrations, which can allow a couple to laugh at themselves – humour often being an important ingredient of marital therapy.

Another aspect of cognitive and behavioural treatments in marital therapy is teaching *communication problem solving*. This will be illustrated in the same couple, where they are in dispute about whether to emigrate to the USA or not:

THERAPIST: This question of whether or not you go to live in the USA is clearly important, and you have told me that you hold opposing views, one way forward might be if you each summarised the *other person's* view on this subject.

RON: She does not want to go because it would mean leaving her friends and family in this country. I also think she might be scared of making the break with England.

MARY: Just like him to make me appear selfish.

THERAPIST: Hang on a minute, neither one of you is responsible for 100 per cent of this problem or 100 per cent of the solution. I want you to try and collaborate to get a solution, so Mary, can you begin by saying what you think are Ron's reasons for wanting to go?

MARY: He wants to give up his job in London, as the pressure is too great. He wants to start his own business in America, and he could join his brother who is already in business out there.

THERAPIST: So it seems Mary has everything to lose, and Ron everything to gain!

RON: No I don't agree. I would also be leaving my friends and some of my family behind, but I do agree that the main gain for me would be to leave that terrible job in London, and I have always wanted to start my own business. I think the business would really succeed there and Mary would benefit financially from that.

As a result of this session each partner felt able to carry out a homework task of writing a list of the *pros* and *cons* of going to the USA. The lists were evaluated at the next session, and some of the most helpful suggestions were mutually agreed. As an example Mary suggested 'If we do decide to go we should find accommodation suitable for my elderly parents to stay with us when they visit, and we should return to England at least once a year.'

The range of problem solving techniques is too large for everything to be included in this volume, but one of the general principals is that the therapist does not just allow 'easy solutions' without proper consideration. For instance the couple were invited to consider a number of 'what would happen if . . .' type questions e.g. 'What would happen if Ron's business venture failed'. At each stage the therapist checked that each spouse could do the thing they had agreed to do, and a progression was made solving minor difficulties until they finally solved the major argument and did decide to emigrate.

At this point it is worth *summarising* the behavioural exchange model:

1   *Positive* rather than *negative* behaviour is emphasised, e.g. 'Stop criticising my appearance' could be translated into 'Say if you approve of my hair or clothes.'

2   *Repeatable* rather than once only behaviour is used, e.g. 'Go to my sister's wedding' is an unsuitable target, but 'Go out socially with me once a week' is acceptable.

3   *Specific* rather than *general* behaviour is preferred, e.g. 'Help me more with the housework' is an over general target, whereas 'Wash the dishes after the evening meal five nights a week' is suitable.

4   It should be *Acceptable* to both parties.

5   It should be *Realistic* rather than overambitious.

6   *Complaints* should be translated into positive wishes.

Case Illustration

Calum and Mhairi Dolan were referred to the clinic due to their GP's concern that Calum suffered from delusional jealousy. They were both in their 30s and had been married for 10 years. The first six years had been happy but the marriage had deteriorated over the past four years following Mhairi being promoted at work. Both of them had previously worked as social workers in the same office but Mhairi's promotion to be a team leader had resulted in her moving to a neighbouring office. Since that time, Calum had been increasingly suspicious and jealous. Their problems at the time of referral had reached the point that both were considering separation but regarded referral to the clinic as their 'last chance of making things work'.

For the first session the therapist allowed the couple to talk freely about their problems for the first hour and a half. At the end of this time, the following hypothesis of their difficulties was suggested:

Assessment

Calum, a quiet and shy man was frustrated in his work. Mhairi's promotion led her to be enthusiastic and on returning home to talk in an animated fashion about her day. Calum could not share her enthusiasm and increasingly made unfavourable comparisons between his own plight and Mhairi's success. The office where Mhairi worked was predominantly male. Calum began to believe that his wife was so happy at work and despondent at home that she must be having an affair. He began quizzing her about her movements and would even phone her several times during the day to check up that she was where she said she would be. This suspicion of Calum was intolerable to Mhairi who began to be evasive in answering his constant enquiries. Calum, therefore, became more concerned and also began feeling resentful and stopped performing his share of household chores. Mhairi had subsequently 'gone off sex' which also increased Calum's suspicions about her fidelity. By the time of referral, Mhairi was threatening to divorce Calum. Both partners appeared to be taking a very rigid stance with the other and their interaction was peppered with insults and arguments.

Treatment

The therapist then asked each of them to think of two tasks each which they would like the other partner to do for the next week. Calum's initial reaction was 'Have sex with me' but it was pointed out to him that this was far too early in therapy to expect Mhairi to agree to such a target.

Mhairi's first target was also unsuitable as she suggested 'Stop quizzing me about my movements'. The therapist explained to her that this would be an almost impossible target for Calum to meet and it would be much better to think of a positive piece of behaviour which was incompatible with the 'quizzing'. To demonstrate this the therapist asked Mhairi when the maximum frequency of 'quizzing' occurred. Mhairi explained that this was as soon as she came in from work. Eventually it was decided that a suitable target was 'To sit next to me when I come in from work for 30 minutes having a cup of tea and discussing topics of general interest, e.g. T.V., films, theatre but *not* work'.

Eventually the following targets for the next week were agreed:

For Calum
1 To sit next to me when I come in from work for 30 minutes having a cup of tea and discussing topics of general interest, e.g. T.V., films, theatre but not work.
2 To wash up the breakfast and evening meal dishes every day.

For Mhairi
1 To cuddle and kiss me at night before going to sleep.
2 To go out with me to the public house, theatre or cinema twice a week.

These targets were written down for both partners. Each was asked, not only to record their own progress but also that of their partner. A further appointment was made for a week later.

At the second session it was immediately clear that things had not gone well. Both Calum and Mhairi looked angry and discontent. Apparently, things had gone reasonably well for the first three days and then Calum had tried to push Mhairi to have sexual intercourse with him when they were kissing and cuddling before bed. Thereafter Mhairi had refused any physical contact with him and this had resulted in Calum also refusing to perform any of his tasks.

The therapist first allowed them to talk about their anger and disappointment. Praise was then given for the initial three days when both partners had achieved their targets. They were then asked if there was any possible way in which they could prevent such a 'mishap' occurring again. Eventually they agreed that they could kiss and cuddle when Mhairi came in from work and before their cup of tea when Calum was less likely to think about sexual intercourse.

These revised tasks were given to them along with another appointment in a week. Over the following weeks, Mhairi and Calum managed their tasks without major difficulties. Additional tasks were added to the list as they felt able to cope with them, and their general relationship improved as they found themselves spending more time together.

After six weeks, they reported that they had resumed sexual relations for the first time in 10 months, and this had occurred at Mhairi's initiative. Calum subsequently began to realise how ridiculous his suspicions were about Mhairi's infidelity. They were discharged from active treatment after eight sessions with the therapist.

The case history of Calum and Mhairi demonstrates how, even apparently complex problems can often be improved by attending to 'minor' issues. Behavioural exchange training has many advantages: it is simple to learn and apply, the therapy is brief, it is goal directed (and can, therefore, be usefully combined with other behavioural treatment packages), and improvement is monitored and measured by both therapist and patient. A number of marital satisfaction questionnaires (e.g. Maudsley Marital Questionnaire described in Crowe, 1978) can also be used to measure progress.

Problems can arise if the couple or one of the partners has poor motivation to change. Unfortunately, motivation is notoriously difficult to assess before embarking on treatment. Most experienced therapists will admit that they have had both pleasant surprises in patients they had felt unmotivated, and unpleasant surprises from those that they felt were highly motivated. One of the best predictors of response is the response to the early sessions. Another criticism of these methods are that they ignore historical issues in a relationship. The standard reply to this has been that historical issues do not matter, or as expressed by Ellis & Harper (1975):

Irrational idea No.8: The idea that your past remains all-important and that because something once strongly influenced your life, it has to keep determining your feeling and behaviour today.

Whereas this dictum may work for most patients with relationship problems, it is certainly untrue for a minority. There is no reason why historical issues need be totally ignored within a behavioural treatment, as the case history of Beatrice and Claude shows.

Case history of a couple where a build up of resentment about past events impeded treatment

Beatrice and Claude were referred to the clinic with a history of deteriorating marital relationship over the past five years. Claude was a managing director of a successful engineering firm, and Beatrice had previously worked as his personal assistant before her marriage, but was currently not in paid employment. They had been married for 15 years, Claude was aged 50 years and Beatrice was 12 years his junior. Beatrice had recently become pregnant with her first child and this appeared to be adding to marital strife.

The first thing that Claude said following the therapist's self-introduction was:

'I do hope you'll be able to help Beatrice, she does have such unreasonable moods and is quite irrational at times. Of course I will do anything I can to help but you must appreciate that I'm a busy man and so won't be able to come here very often.'

The therapist decided not to challenge this statement at this time and started to try and obtain a history from both of them. This proved totally impossible. If Beatrice was speaking, Claude would constantly interrupt *correcting* her on details until she became extremely angry. Claude, on the other hand would only answer questions by referring to 'Beatrice's little problems' which further inflamed his wife. Eventually, it was decided that the best plan was to meet with each of them *separately*, and obtain a personal and marital history in this way.

Claude's interview revealed that, although a successful business man, he had a life-long difficulty in making friends as well as social problems. He was only happy if relating to people he perceived as 'junior' to himself and even then was only relaxed if talking about business matters. At other times, he responded by trying to appear over-confident and realised that he was overbearing. He felt that his wife had gradually stopped loving and trusting him. This belief was based on his observation that she frequently did not tell him what she was going to do until it was to late for him to participate in the decision making. A recent example was that she had organised an amniocentesis appointment without discussing it with him. When asked to focus on possible tasks which he would like Beatrice to agree to he suggested:

1   Discuss with me any decisions made after her antenatal appoint-
    ments, and any decisions to purchase baby equipment before the
    purchase is made.
2   Go out with me once a week to the office social club to meet with the
    other directors and their wives.

Beatrice gave a rather different history. She felt that, although she had originally been very much in love with Claude, he had abused her love. She felt he was over involved with every decision, and even required her to account for every penny which she spent on household goods. Claude not only asked her for details which she felt excessive but also would nearly always disagree with any decision she had made. Because of this problem, she had started to keep information from Claude and to only tell him things if there was no way of keeping it secret. Their social life had stopped as she felt Claude constantly criticised her in public. The tasks she would have liked Claude to perform were:

1   To say at least one positive thing about my abilities for every
    criticism made.
2   To agree to delegate at least one decision a week to me and then to
    leave me to make the decision and to state it without receiving
    criticism and 'advice'.

Following these sessions of individual history taking, the therapist met with the couple and suggested that they consider the tasks that each of them had designed for the other. Both considered the tasks reasonable and acceptable, and so they were asked to record their own and each others progress in achieving them, and were given an appointment in a week.

After two days the therapist received a phone call, firstly from Claude and, later in the same day, from Beatrice. Both reported that they had had a violent argument, and both were refusing to continue to comply with their behavioural tasks. They were asked to try to recommence their programme as well as they felt able, and that a full discussion about the problems would take place in the next session.

At the next session, it was immediately clear that both Beatrice and Claude were extremely angry with each other. Each of them was avoiding eye contact with the other, both were talking simultaneously and trying to 'shout each other down'. Eventually, it was ascertained that during the week, Beatrice had been into town with a neighbour. While in the shops, she had seen a baby bath at a reduced price which she had bought. On returning home, she had told Claude of her purchase. Claude had immediately been very angry as he felt Beatrice had not complied with her task of discussing purchases for the baby with him. He then went on to allude to a time a few months after their marriage when Beatrice had overspent and developed a bank overdraft. Beatrice thought this was unreasonable and countered this accusation by saying that if she had felt able to discuss purchases with Claude without being subjected to 'the Spanish Inquisition' she might not have got into debt in the first place. Following this, there was increased arguing between the couple, mainly about past events. It became clear that so much resentment between the couple had built up over the years that any therapeutic intervention which ignored these historical resentments was doomed to failure.

The therapist, therefore, suggested that they should temporarily abandon their reciprocal tasks and instead a new programme was prescribed. They were asked to discuss with the other all their feelings about events in the past. These were to be tackled in chronological order. No mention was to be made of the other partners 'misdemeanours' but they were to concentrate purely on their own reactions to factual events. To avoid arguments, each was to discuss their emotions for 30 minutes, which should be timed with an alarm clock, after which the other partner's turn commenced. There was a ban on making any reply to or comment on their spouse's emotional reactions. They were asked to do this for a week alternating the order in which they spoke to each other. At the next session, each of them was to be asked to express their partner's point of view and emotional reactions to past events.

At this third session, both seemed more relaxed and cheerful. They both reported that they felt they had already begun to understand each other better. The therapist asked them to summarise their partner's emotional reactions to events at the beginning of their marriage. Both managed to do this well and with empathic appreciation of their spouse's feelings. They were, therefore, given identical tasks for the following week.

After the second week of this programme, they were still proceeding well. The therapist felt it was time to introduce a more interactive style of communication. Beatrice and Claude were asked to continue discussing their emotional reactions to past events, but they could now speak at any time in the daily one hour session. The only stipulation about when they could speak was that the speaker had to hold in their hand a specified object and could not speak if not holding this object. The couple decided that a suitable object to act as a 'mace' in this way was a brass ornament which a close friend had given them as a wedding present. It was re-emphasised to them that the rest of the 'rules' were the same and that each of them was to try to learn the other's point of view. There was still to be no direct retorts to anything that the other partner said. If one of them wanted to speak but the other partner still held the 'mace', they were to signal their desire to speak and then wait until their spouse handed it to them.

The next three weeks were slightly more fraught than the previous few weeks. Generally, they progressed well and had good understanding of their spouse's point of view. Problems arose when they would occasionally speak at times when they did not have the 'mace' but they mostly managed to joke about these occasions. By this time, it became clear that much of the bitterness and resentment had been discussed and handled by Beatrice and Claude. As they had now reached comparatively contemporary events in their discussions, it was time to allow them to talk without the restrictions of the 'mace'. The therapist asked them to still set aside a full hour a day for their discussions. In addition the previously designed tasks were reintroduced into the programme.

Claude and Beatrice progressed extremely well and were able to add in and comply with additional tasks over the next six weeks. At the end of this time, both reported that their marriage had greatly improved and they were discharged from active treatment to follow-up. Before this, Claude asked if the therapist could help him with his social skills problems. Behavioural analysis of the problem demonstrated that although Claude did have some excellent social skills, anxiety prevented him from using them. Therefore, instead of implementing a full social skills package (as described in chapter 7) a programme of *prolonged graduated exposure in real life to the feared situation* was introduced and with most of this done by self-exposure (see chapter 5). Some role-play with video feedback was used for treatment of Claude's tendency to talk loudly about one topic whether or not it interested his listener (see Chapter 7).

Although behavioural exchange training can be usefully employed with the majority of couples with relationship problems, there are some couples whose recurrent communication skills problems lead to resentment and misunderstandings. Most of the work on **communication skills training** has focused on teaching couples *communication problem solving skills* as this appears to be the area where conflicts most frequently arise.

In their training package, Jacobson & Gurman (1986) emphasise that three behavioural techniques are used in communication skills training. These are:

1 Therapist issues instructions of what is required (this may be verbal instruction or via modelling).
2 Behavioural rehearsal, i.e. practice makes perfect.
3 Feedback (verbal, audiotaped, videotaped). NB Positive reinforcement should always be given before any suggestions for change.

The first thing the therapist must do in communication skills training is to ask the couple to discuss something themselves and not to talk to the therapist. The therapist then looks for any 'destructive' communications and makes interventions designed to reduce these. Examples of destructive communications are:

1 Destructive criticism.
2 Generalisation.
3 Mind-reading.
4 Bringing up the past.
5 Putting oneself in the right and partner in the wrong.
6 Logical argument as a weapon.
7 Raising the voice.
8 Using 'the sting in the tail'.

The behaviours which the therapist aims to encourage and replace each of these problem communications are listed below:

1 Express one's own feelings instead of imputing feelings in the other partner or using 'logical argument'.
2 Use specific examples and stick to the point (i.e. do not bring up the past or generalise about matters).
3 Avoid mind-reading.
4 Take responsibility for own actions.
5 Avoid monologues, i.e. say what you need to say and then stop.
6 Examine non-verbal communication.

These rules may sound difficult to remember but are usually easy to spot in practice. Of course, all of us use poor communication skills at some time but with some couples, it is a persistent habit. The following case history illustrates how faulty communication can ruin a marriage.

Case history illustrating the use of communication skills training

Dawn and Montague were referred to the Clinic with a three-year history of recurrent arguments. Both were in their mid-twenties and had been married for seven years. This marriage had been happy until the birth of their son three years ago. Since that time, whenever any decisions needed to be made, arguments would begin. These altercations had been precipitated by relatively major issues such as whether their son should attend nursery school, and also had been precipitated by decisions about where they should go on holiday, the colour of the kitchen curtains, where they should spend Christmas, and even what brand of breakfast cereal they should buy.

A *behavioural assessment* of the problem revealed that the problems only seemed to occur at times when decisions were being made. At other times, both agreed that they had few problems. The therapist asked Dawn and Montague to talk to each other, and to discuss the colour that the kitchen should be painted (an issue cited by them as being unresolved), and the following interaction was noted:

DAWN: I would like it painted white although you would think that was clinical and boring. *(Mind-reading)*

MONTAGUE: White wouldn't look too bad in the kitchen but I'm not happy painting it white after that accident which you had when we were first married – you remember how you poured the strawberry jam down the wall! *(Bringing up the past)* You always are a messy person. *(Generalisation)*

DAWN: Me, messy what about you, you are always spilling things! *(Not sticking to point; generalisation)*

MONTAGUE: Stop being so touchy, you always are at these times of the month. *(Using logical argument)*

DAWN: OH, SHUT UP, YOU SELF-OPINIONATED IDIOT! *(Abuse; raising of voice)*

These types of communication errors were discussed with Montague and Dawn. Alternative answers which were more likely to lead to satisfactory problem-solving were also discussed. The therapist also took an active part in this discussion, modelling appropriate responses and encouraging each to test these out in role play and providing feedback on their performance. After several attempts with faulty communication creeping in again, the following discussion was achieved:

DAWN: I'd like to have the kitchen painted white or a neutral colour like that.

MONTAGUE: White would look very smart but it might get dirty quickly. Magnolia may show the dirt less.

DAWN: I'm not fond of magnolia as it always looks dirty to me. Would it be possible to paint it in a washable paint so that we can wipe it down regularly?

MONTAGUE: That's a good idea, I hadn't thought of that, I shall go to the DIY store this afternoon and have a look.

Instructions were then given to the pair to monitor their own communication, and to stick to the rules of good communication, i.e.:

Express own opinion
Use specific examples

Stick to the point
Avoid mind-reading.
Take responsibility for own actions
Avoid monologues
Watch non-verbal communication

Fig. 8.2. The rules of good communication.

Some of these rules are illustrated in Fig. 8.2.

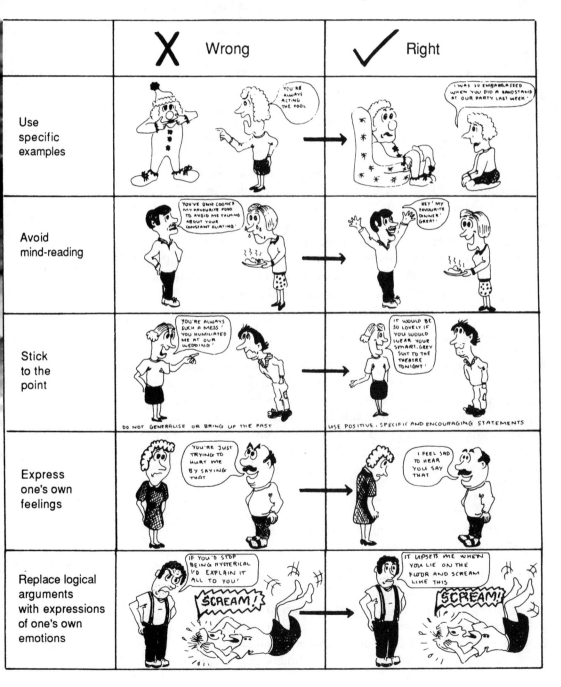

In addition, if any arguments arose, they were to sit down together and examine the type of communication which had been used by each partner, and then practice role-play until a satisfactory problem-solving conversation was achieved. Montague and Dawn were an intelligent couple who grasped the rules of communication quickly, were soon able to laugh at their mistakes, and to correct them. A few further sessions examined the remaining problem areas with them, and they were discharged greatly improved.

Other Techniques

The use of drawings

Not all couples are as receptive, intelligent and insightful as Montague and Dawn. In many cases repeated feedback and role-play by the therapist is needed, and in such cases it is often useful to give the couple drawings of their own most frequent communication errors using their own examples, with more constructive alternatives that are added as therapy progresses. No great artistic skill is needed for this and perfectly understandable cartoons can be drawn with 'pin men' and simple line drawings. This technique not only serves to clearly illustrate the principles which the therapist is trying to teach the couple, but also can add a humorous dimension with the couple laughing at the therapist's attempts at art and even at the ludicrous situations which are depicted.

The use of caring days

Most couples entering marital therapy do not care greatly for each other. However, Stuart (1980) has suggested that if they act *as if* they do care the relationship can improve. The therapist uses the word 'care' rather than 'love' because the former does not have the same mythical and impenetrable qualities as the latter. It is also difficult to encourage people to love each other but perfectly possible to ask them to construct a list of ways each could care for the other. These behaviours must be:

> Positive
> Specific
> Small behaviours occurring at least once daily
> Not the subject of recent conflict

It is suggested that the couple select at least 18 such items, and then each spouse makes a commitment to carry out at least five of the behaviours on the list each day. In this task, each partner is asked to carry out the behaviour regardless of whether the partner has kept his side of the arrangement. The idea behind the caring days technique is that the couple can begin to reverse the often long-standing negative patterns of their relationship, without any apportionment of blame for what might have gone on in the past. Small changes brought about in this way can often be used as an introduction to more fundamental changes in behaviour that were addressed earlier in this chapter.

The role of sex therapy within marital therapy

Some have stated that sex therapy is a specialised subject, and not to be carried out within marital therapy. We discuss sex therapy techniques in detail in the next chapter for the sake of convenience, but our practice is often to *combine* the two approaches. There are many advantages of integrating the techniques: when a couple ask for help with a relationship difficulty and a sexual problem comes to light, if this sexual problem is successfully tackled their relationship usually improves. Much can be done to improve the couples sexual activity by improving communication in general.

Summary

- There are many models of marital therapy but no one model has been shown to be superior to any other.
- There are three main types of behavioural intervention which can be used to help marital or family problems. These are, behavioural exchange therapy, communication skills training and sexual skills training.
- The principles underlying behavioural exchange therapy are: in all marriages each of the individuals adopts behaviours which are the most rewarding and least costly in terms of effort; each of the partners expects a fairly equal sharing of rewards and costs. In problematic marriages this sharing is either unequal or has reached a very low level. This leads to a vicious spiralling of negative interaction and poor control.
- Behavioural exchange therapy is based on definable tasks which are allocated to each of the partners and are performed in a reciprocal or 'give to get' basis. These tasks are designed by the couple with the help of the therapist and arise from wishes expressed by the partners.
- In behavioural exchange therapy the tasks allocated to each of the partners must be: positive rather than negative; repeatable rather than once- only; specific rather than general; acceptable to both parties; realistic rather than overambitious; and complaints should be translated into positive wishes.
- In communication skills training, the therapist asks the couple to talk to each other to identify any faulty communication patterns. These include: destructive criticism; generalisation; mind-reading;

bringing up the past; putting oneself in the right and partner in the wrong; using logical argument as a weapon; raising the voice; using 'the sting in the tail'.

· In communication skills training, the therapist issues instructions of required behaviour which may be a verbal instruction or via modelling. This is followed by behavioural rehearsal and feedback.

9 Sex therapy

The treatment of sexual dysfunction has different origins to most of the other behavioural treatments. Traditionally sexual problems, since the time of Freud, have been considered to be deep-seated neuroses which took many years of analysis to improve. Wolpe (1958) challenged this view by suggesting that systematic desensitisation (see chapter 1) could be used to treat many sexual disorders. Work by Balint (1957) demonstrated that short-term psychotherapy combined with some behavioural techniques could help women with sexual problems, this was also effective for treating male premature ejaculation (Semans, 1956), 'frigidity' (Lazarus, 1963), vaginismus (Haslam, 1965) and erectile dysfunction (Friedman, 1968). However, it was not until the publication of a large study by Masters & Johnson (1970) on behavioural treatment in all types of sexual dysfunction that this became an area of major interest to many health care workers.

Masters & Johnson initially undertook an extensive study of normal human sexual response under a number of conditions, for example different age groups; parity of woman; previous sexual experience; sexual situation, etc. (Masters & Johnson, 1966). Among their findings, perhaps one of the most revolutionary for the time, was that men and women were remarkably similar in the physiological changes which take place during sexual activity. Their four stage model of sexual response is listed in Table 9.1.

Following their discoveries about normal human sexual response, Masters & Johnson (1970) conducted a trial of treatment, based on behavioural methods, for the various forms of sexual dysfunction. This work has been heavily criticised, but the fact still remains that it demolished the Freudian myths about sexual problems. Criticism of their work is generally based on the fact that they advertised for couples with sexual problems in a magazine with a predominantly middle-class readership, thereby skewing their sample to the highly motivated and educated section of society. Secondly, the trial was conducted in a hotel in Florida which undoubtedly produced a 'second honeymoon' atmosphere as well as further excluding those clients who were not extremely motivated as well as well-heeled. Finally, each of the couples worked on their problems for several hours each day, both with their therapists (therapy was performed by two therapists working with each couple) and on their own

Table 9.1. *The four stages of sexual excitement*

Phase	Physiological response	Female result	Male result
1 Excitement	Increase in blood flow to pelvic organs	Vaginal engorgement and lubrication	Penile erection (also requires venous valve closure)
2 Plateau	High sexual arousal; muscle tension and high blood flow levels to pelvic organs	Retraction of shaft of clitoris	Further penile erection
3 Orgasm	Preceded by orgasmic inevitability	Rhythmic contraction of pubococcygeus muscles	Rhythmic contraction of prostate gland, perineal muscles and shaft of penis (leading to ejaculation)
4a Refractory period	————————————————————————		Males only
4 Resolution	Organs return to pre-excitement phase in both sexes. This process is slower with increasing age (and increasing parity with women)		

– a situation which would be impossible for most patients who attend an inner-city psychiatric clinic, where there is already an overburdened service.

Despite the criticism of the scientific merit of their treatment trial, Masters & Johnson produced dramatically successful results which were impossible to ignore. Thereafter, many workers were swept along with a wave of enthusiasm for this new treatment which was then applied by many who knew little about the subject, and by many who believed it was a panacea. Inevitable disappointments followed, but now we know that these techniques can be modified to apply in less ideal settings and can be used to help the majority of patients with sexual difficulties. It has also been shown that there is little advantage in using a co-therapist rather than a single therapist (Crowe, Gillan & Golombok, 1981). The basic treatment package consists of the following steps:

1   Ban on sexual intercourse throughout treatment.
2   Education about sex, basic anatomy and physiology of sexuality, and exploring the couple's sexual vocabulary plus providing a vocabulary for future sessions.
3   Teach relaxation.

4   Non-genital sensate focus.
5   Genital sensate focus.
6   Penetration (initially without pelvic thrusting). This is generally performed in the female superior or lateral positions for most problems except for male retarded ejaculation.
7   Use of different sexual positions and resumption or commencement of full sexual life.

These steps in treatment are demonstrated in the case history of Michael and Lorraine.

Case history of Michael and Lorraine demonstrating treatment of low sexual drive

Michael and Lorraine, both were 23-year-old and had been living together for two years when referred to the clinic with a complaint that Lorraine had never enjoyed sex and would only tolerate Michael's advances to her approximately once every two months. This situation was intolerable to Michael who felt rejected and unloved. Frequent arguments had ensued as Lorraine would refuse any physical contact with Michael fearing it may lead to a sexual advance.

Initially, a full history was taken from each of them. Lorraine, who worked as a primary school teacher had never had any previous sexual experience prior to living with Michael. She was the youngest of six children being raised in a happy and loving Roman Catholic family.

From the age of five years, she had been sent to a Convent girl's school. She had progressed well at this school and had ultimately gained good examination passes enabling her to go on to teacher's training college to take up her chosen career.

She received no sexual education at home, and felt that her parents would have been far too embarrassed to discuss such matters with her. At school the only formal education she had received was from a nun who explained in vague terms that women had to experience 'humiliation' in marriage in order to experience the joy of having children.

Other education which she received from school friends had also hardly been enthusiastic and encouraging about sex. There had been a general belief that sex was a painful and frightening event for the woman who would tolerate it purely for the sake of her partner. Illicit copies of D. H. Lawrence's *Lady Chatterley's Lover* and some pornography which had been smuggled into the school did little to dispel this myth and sex was still generally held to be something which men inflicted on women for their own pleasure.

Her menarche had commenced at age 12 years and had distressed Lorraine greatly as she had not been expecting it, and she found it a frightening and embarrassing event. She had never masturbated as she believed this was 'sinful'. At teacher's training college, Lorraine had met Michael and had started dating him. Their relationship had never been physically passionate although after one year she had allowed him to touch her breasts, but they had not engaged in 'heavy petting' until they had started to live together. She had agreed to live with Michael when she left college but felt guilty about this decision, which was disapproved of by her parents, despite the fact that she no longer felt she was religious. When Michael made any sexual advance to her, she felt 'numb with fear' and wished to end it as soon as possible. She had never been orgasmic.

Michael, also a teacher, worked at a comprehensive school. He had been the only child of elderly parents, had a happy childhood and attended local state schools. Sex had been freely discussed in his household but he still believed that for successful sex the man was responsible for his own and his partner's pleasure. His first sexual experience had been at age 15 years with a girl of similar age that he met at school. This episode had not been enjoyable but he thereafter had had several casual relationships which he had found satisfying. At age 20 years a girlfriend had commented that his penis was small and he had started to worry about this and whether he could thus satisfy any woman. He masturbated twice a week to heterosexual fantasies and had done so since the age of 14 years. The relationship with Lorraine was described by him as being good and close despite the sexual problems.

After the histories of Lorraine and Michael were taken, it was possible to make the following *behavioural formulation:*

> Lorraine has always been brought up to believe that sex is an unpleasant experience for a woman. Therefore, whenever sexual advances are made to her, she expects it to be unenjoyable and nasty. These thoughts lead her to feel anxious and tense, and so instead of being able to relax and enjoy sex, she is constantly preoccupied with her own catastrophic thoughts. This means that sex is never enjoyable to her, which strengthens her negative beliefs, and so the vicious circle becomes complete.
>
> Michael has previously enjoyed sex, but recently has become overly concerned about his sexual performance and ability to satisfy a partner. This means that whenever he starts to make a sexual advance, he is constantly thinking and worrying about his own performance instead of relaxing and enjoying sex. As with Lorraine, these anxieties mean that sex is never fully satisfying and a vicious circle is again formed. Also, Lorraine's present inability to enjoy sex reinforces Michael's feelings of inadequacy.

Both Lorraine and Michael agreed with this formulation. The therapist then explained to them that therapy would be structured to enable both of them to gradually learn to enjoy sex, and would be conducted at their own speed. The ban on intercourse was also explained and imposed. An arrangement to see them in a week was made.

Whereas in most couples presenting with sexual disorders, a full physical examination of both partners is necessary to exclude an organic

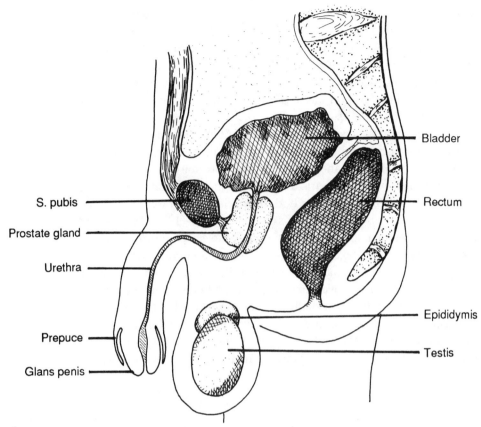

Bladder

Rectum

S. pubis

Prostate gland

Urethra

Epididymis

Testis

Prepuce

Glans penis

Fig. 9.1. The male
genitalia.

Median Section of the Male Pelvis

cause for the problems (for further details of possible organic causes of
sexual dysfunctions see Bancroft, 1983 or Hawton, 1985), in this case the
factors seemed clearly psychological as both had recently undergone full
physical examinations.

In the *second session*, sexual education was commenced. This was
started by using pictures of male and female genitalia (see figs 9.1 and
9.2), and asking the couple to name the different structures and functions, with the therapist giving help when words were not available to
them.

These words that the couple were happy and familiar with were written
down by the therapist so that they could be used throughout therapy. The
therapist then discussed the function and physiology of the sexual organs
and the mechanics of sexual intercourse. Care was taken to correct any
faulty information believed by the couple. For example, it was explained
to Michael that the size of a man's penis had little to do with his ability to
give sexual pleasure to his partner and that in any case, a relatively small
penis tends to enlarge more during erection than a larger one. Michael's

faulty belief that a man was solely responsible for his own and his partner's pleasure was also addressed, as was his idea that a man should always initiate sex. Lorraine's view of sex as something which women were 'subjected to' without personal enjoyment was also challenged.

Relaxation instructions were then given to them (see Appendix 1) and a practice run of relaxation was performed by the therapist together with the couple.

For *homework*, they were asked to set aside one hour a day and to lie on the bed wearing comfortable clothing like night-clothes, in a warm room with soft lighting and gentle background music and to practise relaxation. This was to encourage a hedonistic and relaxed view of their sexual activity. When they were both fully relaxed they were to read an educational book about sex. For this couple Delvin's (1974) *The Book of Love* was recommended as it gives no-nonsense sexual information in a sensitive manner with excellent illustrations. In addition, Lorraine was asked to read a book about women's sexuality on her own (Phillips & Rakusen, 1978). Michael was reminded of the ban on sexual intercourse and told that if he felt very sexually aroused during the homework he was to masturbate. Lorraine expressed interest in this, and said that she would be happy for Michael to do this while lying next to her. The question of birth control was also raised with them and Lorraine admitted

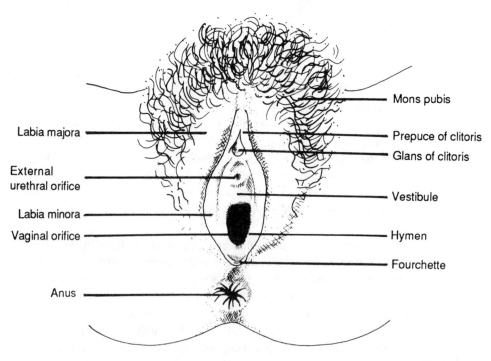

Labia majora

External urethral orifice

Labia minora

Vaginal orifice

Anus

Mons pubis

Prepuce of clitoris

Glans of clitoris

Vestibule

Hymen

Fourchette

Female External Genitalia

Fig. 9.2. The female genitalia.

that this had always frightened her as she did not like to ask the family doctor, who had known her as a child. They were therefore recommended to attend a local family planning clinic together to obtain information. It was agreed that as they had a large amount of homework, they should not meet the therapist again until three weeks later.

At the third session, Lorraine and Michael appeared much more at ease. Firstly, their homework was reviewed with them. Initially Lorraine had been tense and unable to relax but once she realised that she could trust Michael not to attempt sexual intercourse, she had relaxed and found the exercises pleasant and soothing. They had both found the books interesting and useful, and Michael had started reading Lorraine's book. Lorraine had been interested in Michael's obvious pleasure during masturbation and asked if it were possible for her to do likewise. She, however, explained that she did not know how to masturbate. The therapist showed her a picture of female external genitalia which she could take home with her. It was suggested that she might then examine her own genitals using a hand mirror. Then, she could start to touch her genitals and to try to gently rub her clitoris and to insert her finger into her vagina. At all times she should monitor the sensation and continue whatever felt pleasant to her. As she felt unable to do this in front of Michael, it was suggested that she could do this after a warm bath, lying on the bed after she had performed the relaxation exercises (at a time when Michael would agree not to come into the bedroom).

The next stage in therapy was to introduce **non-genital sensate focus**. Michael and Lorraine were asked again to set aside some time every evening when they would not be interrupted by anyone or anything. They were asked again to lie on the bed wearing either no clothes or underwear only. Again the room should be warm, softly lit and with some pleasant background music. After their relaxation exercises, they were to each take turns in touching their partner's body and could do this anywhere except they were *not* to touch each other's genitals or for Michael to touch Lorraine's breasts. This touching should be gentle, and could take the form of rubbing, stroking in circular movements or caressing, and could also be performed with the lips and tongue as well as the fingers and palms. The therapist then asked them to try out these movements with their hands on the back of their partner's hand. Once this was done satisfactorily, the therapist explained that a vital part of the exercise was that the partner who was being fondled should give verbal feedback as to what was pleasant, less pleasant and how they might prefer this to be done. Each of them was to take turns in being the active participant and the recipient. In other words, it was to be performed on a 'give to get' basis with open communication and feedback, to practise discussing sensual and sexual matters freely. It was also suggested that, whereas these exercises could be performed with dry hands, they might also like to try using lotion. Baby oil, body creams and lotions or even KY lubricant jelly were all suitable for this purpose and they were encouraged to try these out and to find which was best for them.

As this is an extremely important step in the treatment which should be performed correctly before moving on to the next stage, an appointment was made to see them in one week.

At the fourth session, the couple reported that they had progressed well. Both were enjoying the non-genital sensate focus and were learning more about what was exciting and pleasurable to their partners and themselves. Lorraine had been shy in giving feedback but this was gradually improving. The therapist praised them for their progress and urged them to continue with this exercise, which was agreeable to both.

Lorraine then asked if she could see the therapist on her own. Michael was happy with this and left the room. She then reported that she had successfully performed self-exploration of her genitals and found this enjoyable. However, she had stopped doing this when she felt that her excitement was increasing as she was not sure what might happen if she 'lost control'. The therapist asked her to think of the last time that this happened and to report what went through her mind at this time. Lorraine reported that she had thought:

I may lose control and go out of my mind.

This thought had immediately caused her to stop the masturbation exercises.

Thus it appeared that Lorraine's negative automatic thought about losing control was severely interfering with her sexual pleasure. The therapist, decided to use a cognitive approach (Beck *et al.*, 1979; chapter 12 of this book) to challenge these thoughts and said:

'Can you think of any evidence to support or refute this belief?'

After much consideration and discussion, Lorraine came up with the following evidence (the figure after each statement is a measure of her belief in each statement rated from 0 = untrue to 100 = absolutely certain).

> *Initial belief*: I may lose control during sexual arousal and go out of my mind; initial rating = 80%
> *Evidence for*:
>
> 1 I feel strange as if I may go mad – 20%
> 2 People in novels do sometimes go mad – 10%
> 3 My cousin had schizophrenia therefore madness runs in the family – 15%
>
> *Evidence against*:
>
> 1 Thousands of women have frequent orgasms and I have never heard of anyone going mad – 75%

2 My friend, Elizabeth, has a schizophrenic brother and is always talking about her sexual experiences – 65%
3 I have seen Michael have orgasms many times without any ill effect – 85%
4 I have got excited about many things and never gone mad – 20%

At the end of this exercise, Lorraine rated her belief that she might lose control and go mad as less than 5 per cent. She was, therefore willing to continue with the self-exploration programme.

The therapist then raised with her whether or not she would be able to discuss her worries in front of Michael, but she felt this would be too embarrassing. Michael was brought back into the room and another appointment made for one week.

When the couple arrived for the fifth session, they both looked cheerful. Lorraine immediately reported that she had masturbated on her own to orgasm. The non-genital sensate focus had progressed well and they had both enjoyed using body lotion in this. The next stage of **genital sensate focus** was therefore explained to them. It is useful for the therapist to be very explicit when explaining this stage as it is important to ensure that the couple understand the exercise, which can also serve as a model for talking about sexual experience without undue coyness. The therapist, therefore, said:

The next stage of genital sensate focus is exactly the same as the previous exercise except that I now want you to include the genital and breast regions. Once again you should start with the relaxation exercises and then to take turns in caressing your partner's body. You may also include the breasts and genitals. The partner who is being touched should tell the other what is enjoyable or how they would prefer this to be done. You can also demonstrate this by guiding your partner's hands and demonstrating what gives you the most pleasure.

Michael, Lorraine will then guide you as to what feels best for her. You may like to start by caressing her breasts and nipples gently and may also use your lips and tongue. Then you could move to the outer and inner labia and try gently rubbing her clitoris and eventually try to insert your finger into her vagina if it is sufficiently slippery and lubricated. You may find that it is even more enjoyable for Lorraine if you gently use your lips and tongue. Lorraine can guide you in this and also in the rhythm and amount of pressure that feels best to her.

Lorraine, you too should try caressing gently Michael's scrotum and penis. The top of the penis is particularly sensitive so be careful to check that you do not press too hard here. You have watched Michael masturbate and so have a good idea of what pleases him but you may like to experiment with other movements and sensations. Again, Michael may find this even more exciting if you also use you lips and tongue.

Michael and Lorraine felt happy with these instructions although Lorraine was unsure as to whether she liked the idea of oral sex. It was explained that this was not mandatory, but that many couples found this extremely pleasant and that they may like to try it even if they decided against it later. A further appointment was made for one week.

When the couple returned they said that they had been successful using the exercises. Michael had been orgasmic on each occasion but Lorraine had not been so yet. The therapist urged them to continue and explained that women were frequently slower to get aroused than men. For this reason it was particularly important that they made sure that the room was comfortable and relaxing, and that the relaxation and non-genital sensate focus exercises were performed first to ensure Lorraine had time to become aroused.

By the seventh session both reported that they had enjoyed several sessions of genital sensate focus, both reaching orgasm and were keen to move on to the next stage. The idea of penetration was then introduced, which should be performed after all the previous steps in the exercises. This was to be carried out with Lorraine in the female superior position, so that Lorraine felt she had greater control. Once both of them felt happy with this, Michael could try some gentle pelvic thrusts, but should stop if Lorraine felt uncomfortable, and then try again when she felt content to continue. After Lorraine and Michael successfully achieved enjoyable intercourse with Lorraine in the female superior position, a repertoire of sexual positions was introduced to add variety into their sex lives. Generally, they progressed extremely well. Lorraine was concerned as she found that she was not orgasmic during penetration although she was during genital sensate focus. It was explained to her that a high percentage of women cannot reach orgasm without additional direct clitoral stimulation during penetration. Despite this fact, she could try by initially commencing penetration immediately prior to orgasmic inevitability and then gradually introducing penetration earlier in the arousal chain. This technique is known as the **bridge manoeuvre** (Kaplan, 1976).

The case history of Lorraine and Michael demonstrates how even fairly deep-seated sexual problems can be dealt with in as little as 10 sessions or 15 hours of the therapist's time spread over four months.

Although the basic package of treatment, illustrated by the previous case, can be used to treat many couples, some specific sexual problems require additional techniques. A list of some sexual problems and their possible treatment approaches is shown in Table 9.2.

Case history of couple presenting with secondary erectile failure

Albert and Maud were referred to the clinic with a seven-month history of Albert being unable to penetrate Maud due to loss of erection. Albert was a 60-year-old dock-worker who had been diagnosed as having late onset diabetes mellitus two years earlier. He regularly attended the diabetic clinic and his condition was controlled by *diet alone*. His erectile problem had started seven months earlier after he had had a week with a lot of overtime. One evening following this, he had tried to make love to

Table 9.2. *Classification of sexual problems*

Stage of arousal	Male	Female	Treatment
Basic drive	Low sex drive	Low sex drive	Basic package (BP) +/− sexual fantasy +/− stop–start technique
Stage 1	Erectile failure		BP + stop–start technique
		Impaired sexual arousal (may cause introital dyspareunia)	BP +/− sexual fantasy or oestrogen cream if post-menopausal
Stage 3	Premature ejaculation		BP + stop–start technique
	Retarded ejaculation		BP – use male superior position for penetration
		Orgasmic Dysfunction	BP + masturbation training programme (if primary dysfunction) May try vibrator if persistent
Miscellaneous	Dyspareunia		Usually physical cause – if not due to anxiety. BP
	Sexual phobia	Sexual phobia	BP + graduated exposure (fantasy + *in vivo*)
		Deep dyspareunia	Change sexual position
		Vaginismus	BP + graded finger insertion or vaginal dilators

Maud but had been unable to penetrate her due to erectile failure. His reaction was one of immediate distress as he was convinced that the problem was related to his diabetes, having read an article in a popular magazine which had mentioned diabetes as being a cause of permanent 'impotence'. Thereafter, whenever he attempted sexual intercourse, he would become anxious that he would fail and this belief was then reinforced by subsequent failure. Prior to the onset of the problem he had enjoyed sex weekly with Maud, both partners being orgasmic.

The first step in treatment was to fully ascertain whether Albert's problem was physical, psychological or a combination of both. It soon became clear on direct questioning that Albert did have an erection during the early stages of sexual arousal, but that this was lost during attempts at penetration. This finding seemed to strongly suggest a psychological basis for the problem which was further evidenced by Albert reporting that he still had normal early morning erections. Although, the evidence seemed to point strongly in favour of a psychological aetiology, a full physical examination was performed to further establish this and also to reassure Albert. This physical examination was entirely normal and showed that Albert's diabetes was well controlled by diet with normal blood sugar levels and no glycosuria.

The next stage in treatment was to start the basic programme of treatment as described in the previous case. Particular tact was needed in the sex education stage as this could easily be seen to be insulting to a couple who had enjoyed a fulfilling sex life for over 30 years. This was achieved by firstly asking them to name the sexual anatomy and functions 'so that the therapist would be using the same words' and then introducing some information about physiology and allowing the couple to ask questions. Once again, *The Book of Love* was recommended for them to read at home as it gives more information than is known by the majority of people.

Maud was unhappy when during the third session non-genital sensate focus was explained to her. She felt that after 33 years of marriage the therapist was treating them like 'young virgins'. The therapist acknowledged that it must have felt like that to her, and then explained that the purpose of this exercise was to re-establish a close sensual and relaxed atmosphere which both partners could enjoy without feeling any pressure to 'perform'.

At the fourth session, the idea of genital sensate focus was introduced but with the addition of instructions for the 'stop–start' technique. This involves asking the couple to caress each others' bodies including the breasts and genitals but once Albert had a good erection, Maud was to stop stimulating him and to allow the erection to reduce a bit before restarting the exercises. They were to repeat this four or five times each session and thereafter, Albert could masturbate if he wished to. The idea of this procedure is to teach the couple that erections can be gained and lost and then re-established again. This removes the type of performance anxiety which occurs with most of these patients who think to themselves, 'Quick, I have an erection I had better use it before it goes'. This type of thinking exerts extreme pressure on the man and usually results in the loss of his erection. Albert and Maud could relate to this suggestion as both of them had noticed that since the ban on penetration had been in force, Albert had a good, strong erection throughout their relaxation and non-genital sensate focus exercises.

This couple, thereafter, proceeded through the programme with good results. At one year follow-up, Albert reported that he still lost his erections occasionally when attempting penetration, but had learnt not to catastrophise this situation, and to resume stimulation either until he regained his erection or, if too tired, to allow Maud to reach orgasm without penetration.

Sexual dysfunction as a result of other factors

The previous two case histories have illustrated how sexual problems may or may not arise in people with predisposing factors, for example strict 'moral' upbringing, faulty or inadequate sexual education, or distressing or traumatic early sexual experience. There is usually, a precipitating event for the problem, for example depression, an episode of alcohol excess, use of drugs, infidelity, ageing, anxiety, emotional reaction to physical ill-health, or childbirth. Finally, maintaining factors can usually be identified, for example anticipation of failure, performance anxiety, restricted sexual skills repertoire, relationship disharmony, or loss of attraction between partners.

Almost any physical illness may result in sexual dysfunction. Even mild influenza will reduce most people's libido and may precipitate a longer standing problem in susceptible individuals. Psychiatric disorder can also frequently result in sexual problems. For this reason the therapist treating sexual dysfunction should be aware of the patient's general mental state, and on their guard for symptoms of depression and anxiety. Although most people are aware of the deleterious effect of large amounts of alcohol on sexual performance, the effect of drugs is often forgotten. As well as illicit drugs, for example heroin which can cause retarded ejaculation, other frequently prescribed drugs including antidepressant and antihypertensive agents, can result in a variety of sexual problems including erectile failure, retarded ejaculation, orgasmic dysfunction and even premature ejaculation. As well as systemic physical causes of sexual dysfunction, the therapist should also be alert to the possibility of local causes, for example imperforate hymen presenting as 'vaginismus', pelvic infection presenting as deep dyspareunia or ejaculatory pain.

Another important precipitating and maintaining factor of all types of sexual dysfunction in both sexes is fear of an unwanted pregnancy. For this reason it is vital to enquire about contraception in all cases and to be ready to provide accurate advice about this where necessary.

Although the two previous case examples have focused on treatment in couples, there are some conditions in which individual treatment may also be required.

Case history of woman with vaginismus

Virginia, a 22-year-old married woman was referred to the clinic accompanied by her husband. They had a two-year history of unconsummated marriage. She had been raised as an only child with parents who were members of a strict Protestant religious sect and had had little or no sexual education. She described herself as totally naive when she married Calvin, her 24-year-old husband. Further details of the history revealed that when Calvin attempted penetration, he felt a marked 'barrier' to his penis entering the vagina. These attempts also seemed to cause Virginia distress and pain and so he had stopped, not wishing to hurt her. Virginia also described a tense feeling in her inner thighs at these times. She had never used tampons for menstruation as, when she had tried, had discovered the same hard ridge which prevented insertion.

The initial step in treatment was to physically examine Virginia to help with the diagnosis and to reassure the couple. This examination must include the attempt at a vaginal examination.

Physical examination of Virginia was normal but attempts at vaginal examination proved impossible, although it categorically established the diagnosis of vaginismus. When the therapist approached the end of the bed, Virginia became tense with an arched back and marked adduction of the thighs. It was impossible to prise her legs apart to any degree with normal pressure.

Having firmly established the diagnosis of vaginismus, the therapist then started by giving relaxation instructions and sex education as in the case of Lorraine and Michael. Again as well as both reading *The Book of Love*, Virginia was also advised to read Phillips & Rakusen's (1978) book, *Our Bodies Ourselves*, on her own. This book gives helpful and easily understandable advice about female sexuality. An appointment was then made to see Virginia alone for the next session.

Traditionally, treatment of vaginismus has been described using the partner from the outset. Although this can be a very valid approach with some couples, the authors have found that better results can often be achieved with very anxious women if they are taught to control their own bodies first before introducing the partner. Of course, some women with vaginismus do present without a partner, having noticed the problem themselves or in previous relationships, and consequently need to be treated alone.

The first session with Virginia alone was used to check that she had understood the sex education and literature which she had been asked to read. Then she was asked to perform self-examination and self-exploration exercises using a hand mirror after having a warm bath, and was relaxed and comfortable without fear of interruption. She was also given instructions in performing **Kegel's exercises**. These are contractions and relaxation of the pubococcygeus muscles. The easiest way to explain these to a patient is to ask them to stop mid-stream while passing urine. Once they can do this, they can try making the same movement when not passing water. If they make this movement slowly, they should be aware that they can contract these muscles to varying degrees. When the muscles are fully contracted, the muscles surrounding the anus are involved and these can be relaxed so that just the anterior muscles are contracting, which in turn can be fully relaxed. The purpose of these exercises in vaginismus is to increase the woman's awareness of the muscles involved in the problem and to establish some control over them.

At the second individual session, Virginia reported some success with the Kegel exercises and self examination, but had not done any self-exploration. She was asked to start self exploration, and to try to monitor pleasurable sensations including trying to gently rub her clitoral region, and to continue anything which was pleasurable. When she was feeling completely relaxed and was enjoying the sensations of touching herself, she was asked to try to gently insert the tip of her finger into her vagina, using a lubricant jelly. While doing this she should try to perform some Kegel exercises a few times and monitor the effect on her vagina. Once she could do this, she was asked to gradually insert more and more of her finger and if she felt able before her next visit, to try with her ring finger and later, her middle finger.

When Lorraine arrived for her next appointment a week later, she reported that although she had managed to insert each of her fingers in turn, she was concerned that this was a 'filthy' thing to do. Further questioning revealed that she still believed that the top of her vagina was 'full of dirty slimy stuff like pus'. The therapist then explained again all about vaginal lubrication and normal female anatomy. As Virginia seemed reassured by this explanation, the therapist asked to continue with the exercises as previously but to try inserting two and then three fingers into her vagina. She was also asked to practise inserting the smallest size of tampon into her vagina and keeping it there for up to two hours (the smallest tampons are those labelled for light menstrual flow).

Three more sessions were needed with Virginia alone, by which time she could happily insert three fingers into her vagina and also insert a medium-sized tampon. Before this stage was reached, a joint session had been held with Calvin and Virginia and they had been started on non-genital sensate focus.

Once Virginia was happy with her ability to insert three fingers into her vagina, the couple were seen and given instructions for genital sensate focus. Virginia was to demonstrate to Calvin how she was best aroused and how to gradually work up to the insertion of his smallest finger. At her own speed, they could move on to larger fingers and eventually more than one finger.

An encouraging sign happened after four weeks of genital sensate focus, when Virginia reported that she had been orgasmic and that Calvin could insert three fingers without causing her pain or distress. The next stage was to move onto penile penetration without movement with

Virginia in the superior position. Once this was achieved, the therapist gave instructions for penetration plus gentle pelvic thrusts and thereafter, alternative sexual positions. The couple continued to progress well with therapy and to maintain their gains at follow-up.

In this case, the therapist used gradual increasing size of fingers to increase Virginia's self-confidence. Masters & Johnson (1970) recommended the use of 'vaginal dilators'. As is clear this is a misnomer as they do not 'dilate' anything and so many people prefer to call them 'trainers'. They consist of glass or, more commonly, plastic rods of graduated diameter which can be inserted into the vagina starting with the smallest. They do have some advantages including their smooth texture which eases insertion, their clear even graduation from one size to the next unlike fingers, and their ability to remain *in situ* for long enough for the woman to get used to them. There are, however, disadvantages including their 'clinical' nature reminding some patients of the doctor's surgery rather than an erotic experience, in addition to their expense. They have a place, therefore, mainly when the use of fingers fails.

The next case example demonstrates how dysfunction in one partner can precipitate dysfunction in the other.

Case example of treatment of premature ejaculation leading to orgasmic dysfunction in the wife

Kelly and Mark were referred to the clinic with an 18-month history of sexual problems. This 22-year-old couple had been married for five years and had initially enjoyed an active and mutually satisfying sex life. Eighteen months earlier, Mark had been involved in a car accident. Although he was not seriously hurt, he was shocked by the event. Two days after the accident, he had made love to Kelly but had found that he had ejaculated within five minutes of starting any foreplay and before he had achieved full penetration. Since that time the problem had continued and had resulted in Kelly being anorgasmic during sexual intercourse.

Mark was convinced that during the accident he had sustained some damage to himself which was causing this problem. He had, however, been fully examined by his GP and referred to a neurologist; all examinations and investigations were normal.

After obtaining the full history, the therapist explained to the couple that it appeared that the road accident had shocked Mark and had lead to a state of high tension and arousal. Although this tension was related to anxiety, physiologically it bears similarities to the changes which take place during sexual arousal. Consequently, when they made love, Mark ejaculated much quicker than usual due to this anxiety. Thereafter, Mark expected to ejaculate prematurely which led, not only to the anticipation of failure, but also to high performance anxiety which resulted in further premature ejaculation. This problem had resulted in insufficiently long stimulation for Kelly to reach orgasm, which had further been complicated by her anticipation of not achieving orgasm before Mark ejaculated and her own performance anxiety.

This explanation was accepted by the couple. Over the next three weeks the therapist had placed a ban on sexual intercourse, had worked with them on sexual education and given them non-genital sensate focus instructions. On the fifth session, the couple were ready to start genital sensate focus. The therapist introduced this in the usual way, giving detailed instructions as to how this could be performed. In addition, instructions were given for Kelly to use the stop–start technique (Semans, 1956). They were given the instruction that when Mark noticed that he was becoming highly aroused during genital sensate focus, he was to indicate this immediately to Kelly who was to immediately stop all stimulation and sexual activity until this arousal subsided which should take no longer than two minutes. They were then to recommence stimulation. This exercise was to be repeated three or four times before allowing Mark to proceed to ejaculation. Mark was to concentrate hard on the sensations in his penis during stimulation and was to signal a level of high arousal to Kelly before reaching the point of ejaculatory inevitability. For the first week, they were to practise with dry hands, but once this was fully mastered, they could try the same exercise with lotion which would increase Mark's arousal as it is a closer approximation to the sensations during vaginal penetration. During genital sensate focus, Kelly was also to instruct Mark as to how he could best stimulate her using his hands, fingers, lips and tongue.

The couple mastered genital sensate focus and the stop–start technique within three weeks. By this time, Kelly was also orgasmic. The therapist then instructed them to move on to vaginal penetration. This was to be performed after the previous steps (with the exception of the stop–start technique which should be used during genital sensate focus only as necessary). Penetration was to be performed with Kelly in the female superior position which results in less concentrated arousing sensations for the man. Once Mark signalled that he was not so aroused that he was about to ejaculate, Kelly was to move, initially gently and slowly and gradually increasing speed, on his penis. Mark was to signal immediately if he was becoming highly aroused and then Kelly should stop all movement until Mark informed her that it was 'safe' to continue. Again, this should be repeated three or four times before allowing Mark to proceed to orgasm.

This couple coped well with the instructions and were soon able to move on to alternative sexual positions and a full and fulfilling sex life. Not all couples, however, cope so easily with the stop–start technique. With some men this technique is insufficient to prevent orgasm. In these cases where the stop–start technique fails, the 'squeeze' technique (Masters & Johnson, 1970) can be used. In this technique, the couple are

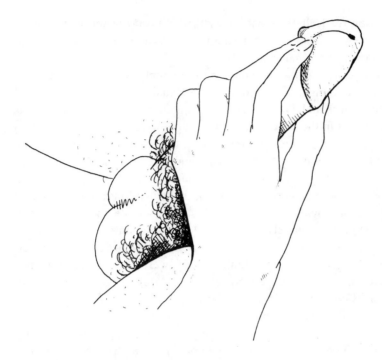

Fig. 9.3. The 'squeeze technique'.

asked to perform genital sensate focus in the manner described above but once the man signals high arousal, the woman is asked to grasp the corona of his penis with her fore and middle finger against her thumb (see Fig. 9.3), applying firm pressure for approximately 20 seconds.

Although this is an effective way of inhibiting ejaculation, it does have the disadvantage of being painful if too much pressure is applied. For this reason some sex therapists have modified the technique from that described by Masters & Johnson and routinely prescribe that the man performs this manoeuvre himself. Whoever performs the technique, the same pattern of practising this three to four times is followed during genital sensate focus before proceeding to orgasm. Once this is mastered, the couple are asked to move on to vaginal penetration and containment as described above.

So far most of this chapter has concentrated on the treatment of *couples*. Some people with sexual dysfunction problems present without a partner. Traditionally, therapists would ask the individual to go away and return once they had a partner. Many of us would feel this is an inappropriately inflexible response. It is difficult enough for most people to start a relationship with a new person without having to also ask them to attend a sexual dysfunction clinic. Obviously the ultimate test for a successful therapeutic outcome, is a mutually satisfying sexual relationship but much can be done in the meantime with the individual to increase their sexual knowledge, their own satisfaction and repertoire of sexual skills.

Case history of Raymond demonstrating individual treatment of retarded ejaculation

Raymond a 30-year-old ex-drug addict, came to the clinic because of his concern that he could take up to one hour during sexual intercourse to reach orgasm. He had no regular girlfriend at the time of presentation but had found this problem extremely embarrassing in the past. He had not masturbated for 10 years, initially because of his reduced sexual interest while he had been using heroin and more recently because he feared that it would 'use up his sexual energy and make me even slower next time I have sex'.

His history was typical of many heroin users. He had enjoyed sex in his teens and had had no problems then. The first involvement with heroin had been at age 20 years at a party but he had found that he soon began to use it regularly, losing his girlfriend, previous social life and job in the process. During the period of his addiction, he had lived rough and turned to petty crime and drug dealing to support his drug habit. At this time he had a girlfriend who was also a drug user. Sex had occurred infrequently due to the reduction of libido produced by heroin and when it had occurred, he had frequently taken up to an hour to reach orgasm.

Five years ago he had been treated for his drug addiction and, after a difficult two years, had obtained a good steady job, non-drug using friends and a flat-share. He had a live-in girlfriend at this time who had left him after one year. It was then that he noticed that he still had retarded ejaculation. Initially, he thought this would improve with time but he became increasingly worried when this failed to occur. For the past two years, he had avoided any sexual relationships for fear of embarrassment because of his problem. He did not masturbate but frequently had spontaneous nocturnal emissions.

Firstly the therapist explained to Raymond how during his period of heroin abuse he had learned that it took him a long time to reach orgasm. Although delayed ejaculation is part of the pharmacological action of heroin, because this lesson was learnt, expectation and anticipatory failure led this to persist even after he had stopped using the drug. In the same way as he had learned retarded ejaculation, he could relearn normal ejaculation.

Next the therapist discussed male sexual anatomy and physiology with him and generally discussed areas of sexual education. He was asked to read a self-help book for men with sexual problems (Zilbergeld, 1980) for homework.

During the second session, instructions in masturbation were given to Raymond. He was asked first to perform relaxation exercises and then to start gently stimulating himself. It was explained that the stop–start technique whereby periods of stimulation were interspersed with a period of stopping stimulation, was usually more arousing. Raymond was also asked to use erotic fantasies to aid his arousal and advised that, if he found them exciting, 'girlie' magazines might increase his arousal at this time.

In fact, Raymond preceded very well with these instructions. To his surprise, he found that once he had relaxed and was in the mood for sexual excitement, he had an orgasm fairly rapidly. He realised that anxiety and anticipation of failure had caused his problem in the past. As there was little else that could be done at this time, Raymond was discharged although asked to re-contact the therapist if he needed to.

One year after Raymond had been last seen in the clinic, the therapist received a letter from him which stated that he was soon getting married, and that he had no other problems since he had realised the role that anxiety played in his difficulties.

Finally, it must not be forgotten that although all the examples cited above have been of couples or individuals with heterosexual orientation, these techniques could be adapted to homosexual couples of either sex.

Summary

- Treatment of sexual dysfunction in a couple can be combined with behavioural marital therapy.
- Human sexual response can be divided into four stages: excitement, plateau, orgasm and resolution.
- Dysfunction may occur in any of the four stages of sexual response.
- The standard treatment for sexual dysfunction begins with *a ban on sexual intercourse throughout treatment*, and is followed by education about sex, basic anatomy and physiology of sexuality, and exploration of the couple's sexual vocabulary plus providing a vocabulary for future sessions.
- This is followed by relaxation training, non-genital sensate focus and then genital sensate focus. Penetration is initially without pelvic thrusting and performed in the female superior position; experimentation with different sexual positions then proceeds.
- Sexual dysfunction techniques may be used for an individual where no partner is available.
- The treatments can be applied to dysfunctions arising in homosexual couples as well as heterosexual.

10 The chronic patient

Patients with obsessive-compulsive disorder or agoraphobia may have suffered for anything up to 40 years or more before presenting for behavioural treatment. However, in this chapter we consider a group of patients where cognitive and behavioural techniques do not necessarily provide a treatment for the basic condition, but where specific techniques may be used to make the patient's or their carer's lives more comfortable.

The role of this type of treatment aimed at reducing undesired behaviours, and increasing socially acceptable behaviour has increased in the past few years with the closure of many of the older psychiatric institutions, and a move towards community care. Discharge to the community or admission to a psychiatric unit of a district general hospital often means that bizarre or socially unacceptable behaviour is not tolerated as readily as in the old 'asylums'. Different problems are also presented by the chronic institutionalised patient, and by the so called 'new long stay' patient, a term to be defined in this chapter.

Firstly, however, we must define *chronic psychiatric disability*. This problem has been addressed by Wing & Morris (1981) who distinguish three types of disability:

1   **Primary impairments**, these are the psychiatric symptoms.
2   **Secondary handicaps**, based on adverse personal reactions as a consequence of having been psychiatrically ill.
3   **Tertiary handicaps**, consisting of social disablements which are either a consequence of the disturbance, or reflect pre-existing factors of deprivation and disadvantage.

In diagnostic terms the primary impairments are, in most cases, the features of schizophrenia, although they may include cases of depression and personality disorder. Much has been written about the secondary and tertiary handicaps, and these are reviewed by Shepherd (1984). These categories emphasise that it is in the area of secondary and tertiary handicaps where behavioural techniques can be applied. The 'new long stay' are new patients who are currently being added to the old long stay population from admission wards and from community follow up. Attempts to reduce the build up of numbers of this category of patient are being done mainly by specialised provision, but also with behavioural techniques.

Many of the techniques to be described are subsumed under the rubric of 'psychiatric rehabilitation'. Rehabilitation has been defined by Bennett (1978) as: 'the process of helping a physically or psychiatrically disabled person to make the best use of his residual disabilities in order to function at an optimum level in as normal a social context as possible'. Rehabilitation can be seen, therefore, as a way to help the patient make the best of what he has in various social roles. The behavioural techniques towards this end can be classified:

1   Operant methods
2   Social and task oriented skills training
3   Behavioural family therapy

Many of the techniques used fall into the heading often described in the UK as 'behavioural modification'. This term is not used in this book, as in the USA the expression is often used to describe the whole of behavioural psychotherapy. Basically we are referring to techniques based on **operant conditioning**, which in common parlance means 'sticks and carrots'. These principles are not always as obvious to apply as on first sight. For a start, one man's stick may be another man's carrot or vice versa. **Premack's principle** (1959) addresses this finding by observing that *high-frequency preferred activity can be used to reinforce lower-frequency, non-preferred activity*. In other words, if a child spends most of his or her time playing with its toy racing cars, this high-frequency preferred activity could be used to reinforce the lower frequency non-preferred activity of tidying his/her bedroom.

By far the most commonly applied form of reinforcement to be used is **positive reinforcement**. **Negative reinforcement** or punishment are hardly ever used, and then only in dangerous or life-threatening situations. The ethical problems with negative reinforcement and punishment are obvious but clear ethical dilemmas may also arise with positive reinforcers, particularly if necessary items such as food are used as reinforcers and the patient has not *earned* a meal that day. The various types of reinforcers are listed in Table 10.1.

In practice *three* main methods are used in changing behaviour in the chronic patient: operant methods, social-task-oriented skills training and behavioural family therapy. These will be illustrated and several examples will be given where operant methods are combined with social skills training as this is widely used in practice.

Case history of woman with urinary incontinence treated by a positive reinforcement programme

Flora an 82-year-old woman had suffered from a cerebrovascular accident two years earlier which had resulted in moderate intellectual

Table 10.1. *Classification of reinforcers*

Reinforcers which increase specified activities

A Positive reinforcers

1 Social approval, e.g. nurse's approval of a patient's improved self-care.

2 Higher frequency preferred activities.

3 Feedback reinforcement, e.g. constructive comments in a social skills group.

4 Food reinforcers.

5 Tokens – awarded for certain activities, which can be 'spent' on a number of other reinforcers.

B Negative reinforcers

This entails removal of an aversive event after a specific response is obtained (aversive relief) but it has little place in contemporary treatment. It may be used covertly in the management of deviant sexual behaviour.

Reinforcers which reduce specified activities

A Punishment

This refers to applying an aversive stimulus in response to certain behaviours. It should have no role in therapy.

B Response cost

1 Penalty involving some time and effort in response to certain behaviours.

2 A positive reinforcer is removed if certain non-desired activities are indulged in. For example, time out (removal of the individual from reinforcing environment for up to 3 minutes). A child who slaps another child is removed from the room for a few minutes.

---

impairment. She had spent the last two years living in a geriatric hospital where her problem of incontinence was a problem to the staff who were required to change her incontinence pad eight or nine times daily. This incontinence was not felt to be organic in origin but attempts to regularly 'toilet' Flora had not produced any obvious success. Despite this, it was noted with interest that Flora was rarely incontinent overnight. The staff found her difficult because of her problem and requested that a behavioural psychotherapist should be asked for advice.

The therapist arranged to spend two days on the ward. The first day was spent observing Flora and obtaining baseline measures for the problem. It rapidly became clear how tired the staff were with Flora's problem and how they had little or no interaction with her except when she was incontinent. The nurses were very busy but were inadvertently reinforcing Flora's incontinence. However, this would not have been useful information for an outsider to impart to the nursing staff after only being on the ward for a few hours, and would have been likely to engender a bitter attitude in the staff. The therapist therefore decided to check how frequently Flora was incontinent by examining her incontinence pad every 30 minutes. In addition, she was taken to the toilet by the nursing staff five times a day as usual. The first day's data revealed that Flora passed small amounts of urine every hour although this was not noticed on every occasion by the nursing staff.

The next day the therapist explained to the staff that Flora was going to be taken to the toilet every 30 minutes. Smiles, praise and social reinforcement would be used whenever she managed to pass water. If she did not urinate, she would be taken back to the day room after five minutes on the toilet without any further communication.

The therapist started this programme as described. At first Flora did not appear to listen to praise when given. This unfamiliarity with social reinforcement was overcome by the therapist looking Flora in the face while smiling and praising at the same time as gently stroking her hand. After four hours of this programme, Flora seemed to understand what she was required to do. She began passing water on almost every visit to the toilet. If wet at other times, this was ignored until her pad was changed at her next toilet visit.

The nursing staff were asked to continue this programme for the next week. Their initial reaction was that they were much too busy to bother with taking her to the toilet every 30 minutes. It was pointed out that the time previously spent in changing not only Flora's incontinence pad, but also the bed on the frequent occasions when overflow occurred, were equivalent. Notwithstanding this argument, most of the nursing staff remained adamant that the task was impossible for them. Luckily, at this point a student nurse spoke out and said that herself and a fellow student could easily take this responsibility on as part of their 'case history project' and that this would work well as they usually had opposite shifts, so that there was only a small amount of time when the rest of the staff had to worry about Flora. It was thus explained to the student how to offer positive reinforcement to Flora and to ignore any incontinence or failure to pass water on the toilet.

When the therapist arrived on the ward a week later, the staff were noticeably more enthusiastic about Flora's programme. It appeared that the general feeling before was that the therapist was some 'clever outsider who's come to show us how to do our job and has just experienced a "flash in the pan" success but is leaving us to do the dirty work'. These attitudes were mellowed to some extent by the continued success of the two student nurses.

The students reported that Flora had not been incontinent for three days but was passing water on each occasion that she was taken to the toilet. The therapist, suggested that they should reduce the frequency of toileting to hourly, and continue monitoring whether her pad was dry or wet, and when she used the lavatory. Only if her pad was wet on more than 50 per cent of occasions for two days should they increase the frequency of toileting to every 45 minutes.

The case history of Flora demonstrates the importance of having a positive attitude to the patient if any form of behaviour change is to be achieved. All too often, busy and demoralised ward staff ask for a behavioural programme for a patient who they do not like. Inevitably this would lead to failure as there would be a temptation to *punish* the patient for his or her misdemeanours and a likely lack of consistency between different staff. It can often be witnessed that the arrival of a new staff member on such a ward can make a world of difference to a patient without any behavioural programme, by purely demonstrating their interest in the patient. In other words **non-contingent positive regard** for the patient is an important prerequisite to any behavioural programme. Clear examples of this truism can be seen in everyday life. If a child is brought up in a loving, caring environment, then the occasional smack or other punishment can be remarkably effective in reducing undesirable behaviours. If a child is neglected, however, smacks and other punishment have little effect on bad behaviour as the child receives attention, albeit negative, which he or she craves almost exclusively in response to being naughty.

Another difficulty which often prevents a behavioural programme from being effective, is that the wishes of the patient are not taken into account. The following case history demonstrates this point.

Case of a man with chronic schizophrenia and poor self care

Fred, a 55-year-old man, had been in hospital for 35 years. He was a popular figure around the hospital, working in the gardens where he took particular pride in his ability to grow the best roses to be seen in the grounds. Although originally diagnosed as suffering from schizophrenia, the main symptoms of that condition were no longer troublesome to him. He had occasional friendly conversations with his 'voices' but found these reassuring and enjoyable. Generally, he was no problem to the ward staff, who over the years had learnt to regard him as a voluntary staff member as he was particularly good at calming down fellow patients who were distressed or disturbed. Fred's main problem was that he had extremely poor self-care and hygiene standards. He would only bath after an argument with one of the staff, and would never think of changing his clothes without prompting. Morning washes involved a member of the nursing staff standing over him until he had been observed to complete the activity.

Fred's lack of cleanliness was no major problem in the hospital ward where the staff were used to cajoling him. However, the hospital was due for closure in 10 years' time and steps were being made to identify patients who could be discharged to group homes in the community. Inevitably, Fred's pleasant personality, lack of disturbing symptoms and the staff's desire to see him settled in a warm, friendly environment rather than transferred to another long-stay ward, meant that he was one of the first patients suggested for rehabilitation with a view to transfer.

The group home to which it was hoped to transfer Fred was for eight patients who required little staff support in a neighbouring town. Although there were to be two staff members there during the day and domestic staff, as well as visiting social workers, occupational therapists and psychiatrists, the home was not staffed overnight. This required that the patients should all have a high level of functioning and be essentially self-reliant and responsible for their own self-care and cook their own breakfast and supper. Fred, along with the other patients considered for transfer were taken to visit the home. Thereafter, occupational therapy assessments were made as to their domestic abilities.

Fred had never had to cook or care for himself and thus an intensive cooking and home management course was arranged for him by the occupational therapy department. Unfortunately, this reduced the amount of time that he could spend in the hospital gardens. In addition, a behavioural programme was set up so that certain items of self-care were rewarded by time which he could spend gardening. The programme for the first week was as follows:

Fred was to be accompanied by a staff member throughout the self-care procedures, and each step in the programme was to be awarded the following points, *only* if the staff member had to prompt Fred not more than twice *without* argument.

After breakfast

Go into the washroom	1 point
Fill wash basin with water	1 point
Wash hands and face	3 points
Dry self with towel	2 points
Clean teeth	5 points
Use electrical shaver	5 points

After supper

Go into bathroom	2 points
Run bath	2 points
Climb into bath water	2 points

Soap and wash following:

Right leg	3 points
Left leg	3 points
Right arm	3 points
Left arm	3 points
Front torso	3 points
Back torso	3 points
Neck	1 point
Face	2 points
Use towel to dry self	4 points
Clean teeth	5 points

Maximum possible number of points = 53

In addition if Fred washed hands after using toilet, before meals or after soiling hands in garden, he should be awarded three points on each occasion.

Each point can be redeemed for the privilege of spending one minute in the hospital garden to be taken at time agreed by Fred.

Progress with this programme was to be recorded by the nursing staff. The programme was shown to Fred himself, so that he was aware of the behaviours required of him to earn his rewards. The first week of this programme proved a failure. Whereas the initial programme had been geared so that Fred, on the basis of his previous performance, was likely to earn at least 45 minutes in the garden a day, he now earned less than five minutes a day. Previously he had required few prompts to wash, but now needed seven or eight prompts for most activities. At the end of the week, his behaviour had deteriorated further, he had been irritable when asked to wash, and on one occasion had tried to punch a male nurse who had asked him to get into the bath. Fred had not been known to be violent before. In addition, he was refusing to attend the occupational therapy programme.

The staff decided to make the programme easier. It was decided to double the point system, and to only prompt him twice for any activity, and thereafter if he had not performed it, to forget about it. During the second week he deteriorated further, and was rarely washing at all. He had also been incontinent of urine on three occasions in the patients' lounge, an event previously inconceivable to the staff.

A team meeting was then held to which Fred was invited. After some prompting, Fred expressed extreme anger at the way a programme had been introduced which restricted his access to the garden. He did not want to be discharged or as he said, 'sent away from my home after so many years'. In addition, he had noticed that the group home had no garden and felt he would be 'banished to a life without my main pleasure in life'. After much discussion and consideration, it was decided that Fred should not be transferred to the new group home. It was explained to him that the hospital would definitely be closed down in the future, and that everyone could understand how angry and miserable this must make him feel after being there for so many years.

Six months later a second group home was being planned. Fred was invited to look at this and was asked his opinion about it. It had a large garden, and he was promised that if he moved there he should be given his own vegetable garden, as well as being able to look after the flowers. Fred was much more enthusiastic about this home particularly as one of the staff members from the ward whom he particularly liked was also transferring there. After some consideration, Fred agreed to go. This time he needed no prompting to attend occupational therapy, and much to the staff's surprise, his self-care improved dramatically as he became more increasingly impatient to move to his new home. No behavioural programme was needed as Fred himself said, 'If I want to do something I usually can'.

Fred's case raises some of the ethical issues which may be involved in any programme aimed at altering behaviour in adults. Wherever possible, it is important to try and work towards the same goals as the patient and to discuss the issues fully with them. In some patients, however, the ethical issues are quite clear.

Case history of Polly demonstrating treatment of violence

Polly, a 45-year-old chronic schizophrenic patient had been managed at home for many years by her unmarried brother. Admission to hospital had been precipitated by her unprovoked violence towards certain strangers. Although she had always had this tendency, her brother had been able to cope. However, over the past few years, Polly had gained weight, and this combined with her brother's increasing age had led to his inability to prevent her aggressive onslaughts.

Polly would refuse to answer any questions about her violent outbursts and would sit looking at the floor, mumbling unintelligibly when asked about them. Although she was usually friendly to people, observation of her behaviour on the ward demonstrated that she would suddenly lash out at strangers who were smaller than herself. Generally, it was possible to predict when Polly would be aggressive, as she would appear irritable on that morning and pace around glaring at people before the attack. Her victim was usually someone who tried to speak or moved close to her at this time. After she had begun to attack, the staff would physically restrain her. These episodes occurred once every three or four days. When at home, if she was in a bad mood her brother would try to 'cheer her up' by cooking her favourite meal of bacon and eggs.

Polly generally enjoyed attention from other people and liked to go out to the shops and on outings away from the hospital. It was decided to use both of these as positive reinforcers for her behavioural programme. As no predictors for her 'bad' mornings could be found, it was decided that when Polly was in an angry mood, she should be left alone by the staff. Any attempts on her part to engage staff in appropriate conversation at these times would be rewarded by the staff member allowing her 10 minutes of their time. During the rest of the time she would be allotted three 10 minute periods of one to one conversation with a staff member every day and would go on outings daily. Any violent outbursts meant that she lost the privilege of all one to one discussion with staff and the outing for the next 24 hours. Her progress was monitored by staff, and recorded on charts to ensure consistency between staff members, and to guarantee that the information was passed on. Polly was informed in detail about the programme.

The programme did not proceed without hitch. An initial problem was ensuring that staff actually did record her progress. Secondly, consistency was a problem, as some staff would feel they did not wish to stop their 10 minute conversations with Polly even if she had been violent as they believed it to be cruel. Thirdly, some staff would record any irritability as an episode of violence, whereas others would choose to ignore minor physical attacks. These problems were gradually overcome by explaining the importance of consistency to the staff. The idea that the programme was cruel was discussed, along with the question of whether it was not even more cruel not to treat her, and to leave her in long-stay hospital accommodation rather than controlling her behaviour with the view to discharging her home to her brother.

Eventually these staff difficulties were overcome, and the programme was applied consistently. Over the next few weeks, Polly's behaviour improved dramatically, and the next stage was to try to ensure that the behavioural change would continue in her home environment. This can be a shortfall of reinforcement programmes as frequently the improvement will only last as long as contingent reinforcement is in operation. In many cases the outside world does not offer predictable positive reinforcement in response to good behaviour, and the gains of treatment are lost. In Polly's case, however, her brother would be at home with her, and so the training offered a good chance for the continuation of the programme.

The key worker from the ward visited Polly's brother at home. The first thing suggested was that Polly was not offered her favourite foods whenever she was irritable, as this could contribute to the problem. Indeed, Polly had been overweight on admission to hospital but a well-balanced diet had resulted in her achieving a suitable weight for her height. Dietary advice was given, and it was suggested that Polly should only be allowed her grilled bacon and eggs for breakfast if she had not been aggressive the previous day. Similarly, daily outings should be contingent on her non-violence. It was more difficult to continue a programme of rigid times for Polly to receive attention from her brother but it was suggested that if she did appear irritable, he should leave her alone unless she initiated appropriate conversation with him. Although these instructions were superficially simple, habits of a lifetime would be hard to break, and the therapist elaborated examples of Polly's possible behaviours, and suitable responses from her brother in detail. In addition, the therapist practised some of these situations with Polly's brother using role play.

Following this visit, Polly was allowed home for a week's leave. The therapist visited them during this week and her brother was instructed to contact the ward immediately if any problems arose that he could not handle. The week generally went well and Polly was discharged home. Arrangements were made for close continued contact with them via a community psychiatric nurse, who was informed in detail about the programme, as well as frequent clinic visits. Polly is still occasionally violent but her brother can now cope with her and they remain happily in the community.

Polly's case history illustrates the importance of continued involvement with a chronic patient following discharge from hospital if any hope of continued maintenance of gains is to be achieved.

As can be seen from the above examples, in chronic schizophrenia, the main focus of therapy is on the *deficit* aspect of the disorder rather than altering specific patterns of unwanted behaviour, as is done in personality disorder. The *pace* of treatment is slower and the goals of the therapy are more limited. Treatment is directed at one goal at a time, as the patient with schizophrenia finds it difficult to successfully process more than one stimulus at a time. In addition, there has to be **over-learning** of each of the behaviours, to make sure the gains in treatment are not lost later on.

The case of Daryl illustrating some of the problems of badly constructed, inappropriate, or 'amateur' reinforcement programmes in a boy with severe learning difficulties

Daryl, a deaf, blind and mute boy of 15 years with severe intellectual impairments, lived in a local authority children's home. He was a tall boy, being over 6 feet in height which caused the staff some difficulties when they tried to restrain him if he was doing anything dangerous. Nevertheless, they had coped well with him and demonstrated a loving and caring attitude toward him.

Over the previous six months, however, Daryl had developed a new behavioural problem that was causing great concern to the staff. Initially, he had discovered masturbation which had caused few problems, as the staff would remove him to his own room whenever he began to masturbate in a public place. However, Daryl seemed to increase the frequency of masturbation over the next few weeks and was currently masturbating 15 to 20 times a day. The consequence of this problem was that he had been banned from his training centre, as his behaviour distressed the staff who were concerned about the reaction of the parents of the other pupils. He also was unable to go on outings with the Home as there had been complaints from the public about his behaviour.

One of the staff members, Anne, had read about contingent reinforcement programmes and decided to try and implement one with Daryl to reduce his masturbatory behaviour. Anne decided that as Daryl enjoyed eating chocolate beans, these could be used as reinforcers. Every 15 minutes, staff were to check on Daryl and if he was not masturbating or if he was masturbating in his room, he was to be given a chocolate bean. This programme was applied for three months before the staff admitted defeat and requested help from a behavioural psychotherapist.

By this time, Daryl was not only masturbating as frequently as before, he had also gained a considerable amount of weight which meant that it was almost impossible to restrain him when he did start masturbating in public. It was explained to the staff that the reinforcement programme used was not ideal for two main reasons. Firstly, it would inevitably lead to Daryl becoming obese and secondly, chocolate beans were clearly not as rewarding as masturbation to him.

An alternative programme was suggested by the therapist. This involved using masturbation (*a high frequency preferred activity*) to reinforce periods of appropriate social contact. In other words, Daryl was allowed to masturbate on his own for 10 minutes for every hour in which he did not indulge in this in public. Staff were to initially ensure this by holding his hands whenever he was in a public place. As Daryl would need rapid reinforcement for any behaviour, it was arranged that he could not only be taken to his own bedroom, but there would also be a quiet room available for him at his training centre, and he could retire to a corner of the minibus when on outings. This programme was much more successful, and soon staff no longer needed to hold Daryl's hands in public, as he would wait until he was alone. Any relapse required a staff member to firmly take Daryl's hands away from his genital area, and hold them firmly for 10 minutes, which was an activity he disliked.

A case history demonstrating the successful rehabilitation of a chronic schizophrenic patient with multiple skills deficits

Joan was a 45-year-old woman whose medical treatment for a chronic schizophrenic illness had been completely successful. She had lost all the florid psychotic features such as auditory hallucinations, but remained all day shut in her room, living the life of a recluse. She lived at home with her elderly parents and had not worked for many years, although in the past she had trained and worked as a pastry cook. She was treated for a short time in hospital, and this time was kept to a minimum to avoid the dangers of *institutionalisation*, however it was soon clear that Joan was institutionalised in her own home in the sense that everything was done for her by her parents, who said:

> If we don't feed her she will simply starve, she has no idea of looking after herself and can't even boil an egg. If we don't wash her clothes and replace them when they need it, she will smell and look like a tramp.

Additional problems for Joan to become more socially acceptable were that she rarely spoke because of her lack of conversational skills, and she stared at people or never listened to other people if they spoke to her.

Assessment

Joan's problems were broken down into the three categories that commonly are the main difficulties in chronic schizophrenia:

1   Practical skills deficit
2   Conversational skills deficit
3   Social perception deficit

Treatment of practical skills deficit

Three main techniques were used:

1   **Coaching**
2   Rehearsal
3   Praise

The use of coaching to teach new or lost skills

The therapist visited Joan at home and decided to concentrate on teaching her:

1   How to wash her clothing, both by hand and by using a washing machine.
2   How to cook simple snacks.

The therapist simply showed her how to carry out these procedures breaking them down into simple easy steps, for example washing out underwear was demonstrated and the patient was asked to copy this. After some practice she was able to carry out this task and soon afterwards learnt to master the washing machine. She needed a great deal of *rehearsal* before she was able to wash the clothes herself and *praise* was essential to increase her confidence. Her parents had to be told that she could cope, and had to be prevented from sabotaging the treatment until they realised that Joan would come to no harm and she would not wreck the washing machine.

The use of rehearsal in rehabilitation

Rehearsal means doing things again and again! Anyone who has taught a skill to their child knows the importance of this in learning new behaviour. Joan was coached to cook a simple snack and seemed to understand what was required fairly easily in that she could copy each action of the therapist, and with the therapist at her elbow had no problems. However, without the therapist there she would do such things as put an egg on to boil with no water in the saucepan.

'You put in the egg, then you put in the water, *then* you put the saucepan on the stove' were the instructions she had to repeat to herself time and again.

This technique is very tedious to carry out, as all parents of young children know. For this reason rehearsal is often carried out by several therapists working in conjunction in a setting such as a day centre.

The use of praise in rehabilitation

Joan was told: 'You are looking very nice today, I like that new sweater you bought' or 'your new hairstyle makes you look very attractive'.

Praise is something we all like to have and is used to shape behaviour in rehabilitation.

Treatment of conversational skills deficit

Many of the techniques described in the chapter on social skills training (chapter 7), can be used here, for example practice with feedback using videotapes, although techniques are more often focused on more basic skills. These involve:

1   How to start a conversation.
2   How to maintain a conversation.
3   How to end a conversation.

In order to help her start and end a conversation, Joan was taught some simple 'recipes' for success: her previous training as a pastry cook was used to provide a model for how putting simple things together could make something, in this case conversation. She was taught to use appropriate greetings such as 'Good morning', 'Good afternoon' and 'Good evening', and practised these with her therapist. The therapist suggested some opening conversations such as 'I see it has been raining', ' Do you mind if I watch TV with you?' etc., and after practising with the therapist she tried these phrases on her amazed parents. The parents were surprised because she had not had a conversation with them for years. Ending conversations was also taught, and *practice* and *coaching* used with such phrases as 'It must be rather late, I really should be going to bed soon'.

Maintaining conversations was especially hard for Joan. To help with this she was taught the difference between *open-ended* questions such as 'Have you seen anything interesting on TV recently?' which serve to encourage general conversation, and *close-ended* ones 'Is my supper ready?' which do not. Her parents were also taught to give social reinforcement for her conversational skills, by saying such things as 'It is really nice to be able to talk together'.

Other non-verbal factors (eye contact, expressive tone, speed of speech, etc.) are also important, and were taught here in a similar way to the case of Jeffrey (see chapter 7).

Treatment of social perception skills

When her practical and conversational skills had improved there was still something 'rather odd about Joan' as her parents put it, and those who met her agreed. Patients such as Joan are often *irrelevant* in the things they say and this is part of the problem. For instance Joan would talk to her parents or their friends about her menstrual cycle, and details of hallucinations experienced long ago. She needed to learn that it was more appropriate to mention these things to the community psychiatric nurse when she visited. She also had to be taught the value of *listening*. Joan would often cut across other peoples' conversations as she was so involved in her own world that it was often difficult to attend to others. The inability to listen to others is a serious social handicap, as if the information taken in is inaccurate the responses are likely to be inappropriate.

Another difficulty in this area is *perception of emotions* in others. After there had been a death in the family her parents showed their grief by looking sad and dressing in dark clothes. Joan 'let the side down' by playing loud music in her room, and not responding to the obvious emotions of her parents with sadness of her own. She was given some coaching in how to interpret emotions in other people, but this was probably the least successful aspect of the therapy.

After some months of these techniques, Joan learnt how to dress and look after her own clothing. She could shop for herself and cook a simple meal, and if people saw her in the street they did not notice anything abnormal about her. She could have a conversation with people she knew such as her parents, and they considered her to be vastly improved despite the fact that at times she 'let the side down'. After intensive sessions in her own home she attended a day centre, and went on from there to a sheltered workshop. Here she learnt to practise again some of her lost cookery skills and helped out in the canteen.

Despite this apparent success, Joan's favourite activity was watching television alone in her room. What is wrong with that, many might say. She had received social skills training in a wide area, in addition to coaching and rehearsal for self-care and cooking skills, but her overall social skills remained limited. She was unable to learn how to initiate conversation, and she never succeeded in making new relationships. In many cases only limited gains can be achieved, and it is so far not possible to predict how far treatment is going to succeed.

Application of these techniques to people with severe learning difficulties

Many of these techniques can also be used to help people other than the adult mentally ill. The realms of skill acquisition in those with severe learning difficulties is a highly specialist area which is outside the realms of this book. However, contingent positive reinforcement can be used to teach these children and adults a range of skills including self-care and speech. Normally, the reinforcement needs to be immediately after the desired response as many of these individuals have a limited capacity to anticipate and wait for reward. The use of reinforcement is generally graduated to each step towards the goal behaviour. For example, if teaching a child to feed herself, the therapist may first reward the child touching the spoon and then once this is mastered, move on to only rewarding picking up a spoon. In rare life-threatening situations, when positive reinforcement for more desirable non-dangerous behaviours has failed, **punishment** or negative reinforcement may be tried with these children. For example, a 6-year-old severely disabled boy hit his head on walls and on other hard objects to such an extent that he suffered further brain damage. Attempts to divert and reward him for behaviours other than head-banging had failed. Even putting him in padded surroundings had problems as it led to his isolation from all but his key-workers. In the light of this, it was decided to introduce a technique of covering his eyes and ears with pads for 60 seconds every time he engaged in this activity. As he enjoyed watching and listening to the other children this was a form of punishment (*time out from positive reinforcement*). This significantly reduced the amount of head-banging activity, so that he could be managed with the other children rather than on his own in a padded environment. The eye and ear covering had to be repeated at intervals, however, to maintain this reduction.

Ward or group-based behavioural treatments

So far all the case histories described, have featured individual pro-grammes. However, frequently they need to be applied in ward-based settings or with groups of patients for issues of cost-efficiency.

Ayllon & Azrin pioneered one such ward or group-based programme in the form of token economy systems (Ayllon & Azrin, 1968). The idea behind this was that individual target behaviours and problem areas were identified for each patient as well as a reinforcement schedule. Instead of the usual reinforcers, tokens were given as rewards in response to target behaviours. These tokens could then be exchanged by the patient for a number of rewards, each of which had a certain token 'price'. The rewards used included a single room, food, cigarettes, outings and even, on occasions meals (if a meal was not earned, a liquid meal substitute being given). The initial claims for token economy systems were ambitious, and it was tried with groups of chronic psychiatric patients, institutionalised mentally handicapped adults, and children with severe learning difficulties with *apparently* miraculous results.

A controlled evaluation performed in the UK, however, threw some doubt as to the efficacy of tokens *per se*. Hall, Baker & Hutchinson (1977) performed a controlled trial in a hospital in Wakefield. Taking chronic schizophrenic patients who had been continuously in hospital for at least two years, they matched them and randomly allocated them to one of three wards. The 'experimental' group were admitted to the token economy ward where there was a highly motivating environment with new staff and many activities in addition to the token economy. Another group was moved to a control ward where the same highly motivating and stimulating environment with new enthusiastic staff existed. A third group remained in a traditional chronic ward. It was found that whereas the introduction of tokens had an initial effect on target behaviours, this was not sustained. Both active rehabilitation wards resulted in greater improvement in negative symptoms and more discharges to the community than patients from the chronic ward, although this was at the expense of a slight increase in positive symptoms of schizophrenia in the stimulating environments. Interestingly, although this study failed to demonstrate the efficacy of tokens themselves, the nursing staff involved in the study requested that the system should be continued at the end of the research as they found the structure and their ability to reward certain behaviours useful.

The above research has been described in some detail as it raises a number of vital clinical issues. Firstly, it demonstrates the importance of an enthusiastic and fulfilled ward-based staff, if behaviour change is to be achieved. This emphasises the need for maintaining staff morale and the introduction of 'new blood' from time to time to 'fuel' the enthusiasm. Secondly, a moderately stimulating and interesting environment was beneficial to the patients. Thirdly, the structure and ability to reward patients was seen as valuable and important by the ward-based staff. The apparent success of good token economy systems may be the result of the effect on morale which they have on ward staff. The disadvantages of tokens are that they are sometimes a difficult concept for patients to grasp, and many people working in this field prefer to use more tangible reinforcers such as money.

Treatment of schizophrenia of recent onset

So far this chapter has concentrated on the problems of chronic patients in institutions. Nowadays, attempts are made, wherever possible, to return an individual to the community following an acute relapse of schizophrenia. The role of drugs in preventing relapse is not in question, nor is the vital part they play in acute schizophrenic episode.

Recent research has examined the way families cope with a schizophrenic member and the possible effect of family interaction styles on the frequency of relapse in that individual (Leff & Vaughn, 1985). The importance of the level of **expressed emotion** (EE) in a family member in determining future relapse in a schizophrenic patient is being recognised. It appeared that a schizophrenic patient who was discharged home to an environment where at least one family member appeared frequently to express emotional reactions (either positive or negative) to the patient, was more likely to experience rapid relapse of his/her psychotic state than a patient returned to an environment with low expressed emotion.

Initial reaction to this finding was to find alternative placement for patients who had lived in high EE families before their acute episode. Clearly this solution raised a number of ethical, political and social questions. A more positive approach to this problem has been to provide help for the families of schizophrenic patients to cope with the patient, and to use specific techniques aimed at reducing high EE in those families where this is appropriate. EE has been shown to have two main components: **over-involvement** and **criticism**. Over-involvement means over-protective or over-concerned behaviour out of proportion to the realistic needs, and criticism means high levels of derogatory or disapproving remarks, usually related to something that the relative felt had always been part of the patient's behaviour and that they always disliked.

Several books have been written on this subject and only a brief résumé can be given in this chapter. For more detail of behavioural family treatment the reader is referred to Falloon (1985), and Shepherd (1984). The treatment programme involves: education of the family about schizophrenia, support and specific techniques. Each of these will now be separately considered:

Education of the family about schizophrenia

Detailed information is given about topics such as the nature of the disorder, its prognosis and treatment, and research into the genetics and biochemistry of schizophrenia. This clearly needs to be given at a level that is comprehensible to the relatives. Written literature is also often given to back up this information. This information can often most economically be delivered to groups of relatives. The disadvantage is that those who may not understand the information may feel inhibited in asking questions and also the speed at which information is given has to be aimed at the slowest member of the group. The advantage, however, is the support that the families can get from each other as well as from sharing information.

Support

This needs to take several forms. Psychiatric support is needed in the form of access to advice which can be obtained immediately as well as 24 hours a day. Support with medication and practical psychiatric help is probably best provided by the community psychiatric nursing service. Other professional help includes social work, day centre activities and occupational therapy for the patient. In addition, mutual support from families in similar situations is extremely helpful to most people.

Specific techniques aimed at altering communication

If the family has a member who demonstrates high EE, steps can be taken to alter this. This is done by a combination of education, role play, modelling and feedback. Family therapy is a complicated subject with a variety of theoretical frameworks. One approach (e.g. Falloon *et al.*, 1984) involves offering the family basic information about schizophrenia, and also information about the services that are available. Helping the families of patients with schizophrenia to keep some kind of distance from the patient – something that is easier said than done – is thought to be helpful. Towards this end Kuipers (1979) suggests a number of rules for the relatives:

1   Set clear rules and standards
2   Coax sympathetically, but don't pressure
3   Know when to ignore
4   Don't argue with delusions, accept their subjective reality, while not necessarily agreeing with their objective truth
5   Use distractions
6   Use humour (occasionally)

Rather than any strict family therapy technique a general 'family approach' is advocated. This implies a willingness to talk to families, and to listen to their problems, using the kind of general rules outlined above. Some of the problems, and the techniques that can be used to solve them will be illustrated in the next case.

Case history of Ralph, a schizophrenic man with an overdependent relationship with his mother

Ralph, a 36-year-old man lived at home with his elderly mother. His 40-year-old sister, Mary, lived nearby and visited daily. Over the last 10 years, Ralph had suffered from acute relapses of his psychotic state, which occurred yearly. At other times he had no obvious psychotic symptoms but was withdrawn and would socially isolate himself, preferring to spend hours away from the house indulging in his hobby of train spotting.

Once the mother and sister were interviewed with Ralph, the hostility of Mary towards him became apparent. Ralph's father had left home when Ralph was 10 years old. He had been an alcoholic who had frequently been aggressive to his wife and the children. Mary felt that Ralph 'took after' her father and felt that his condition was in some way due to his being weak-willed. His mother was more ambivalent. On one hand she would treat him as a child, insisting on supervising his self-care, making his bed, providing his food and insisting on knowing about his every movement and even reading any letters he received. On the other hand, she was frequently irritable and critical of him as she also felt he was lazy and 'lacked moral fibre'.

Initially the therapist asked the family what they knew about Ralph's condition. It soon transpired that they knew very little, and could not even understand the diagnosis. They knew that he received fortnightly injections of medicine at the clinic but were uncertain why. The therapist started by giving some basic information about Ralph's condition, allowing them to ask questions at each stage. Further appointments were made for this purpose but, in addition, the therapist urged them to contact an organisation for mental illness sufferers in the UK called MIND, and to attend their meetings. After three further meetings with the therapist, the family were well informed about Ralph's condition and Ralph himself reported that 'they don't get on at me quite so much'.

Nevertheless, the therapist noted that his mother still oscillated between treating him as a child and being hostile towards him, although Mary appeared to have become more tolerant. The therapist, therefore, asked the family if there were any remaining problems and any difficulties in coping with each other. Ralph's mother said: 'Well, I really wish Ralph would go out and get a job, he's so pathetic sitting around at home. Any real man would go and get himself a job, but I suppose I shall just have to make allowances for him not being normal'.

The therapist replied: 'I can understand how frustrated you must feel, but I wonder if the way you expressed your frustration might not be rather hurtful to Ralph as well as being untrue. What do you think Ralph?'

No reply was received from Ralph who spent the time looking at the ceiling and intermittently muttering to himself. The therapist therefore started to discuss rules of effective communication with the family. These were essentially along the same lines as those discussed in chapter 8, i.e.:

1   Express one's own feelings instead of imputing feelings in another family member or using 'logical argument'.
2   Use specific examples and stick to the point (i.e. do not bring up the past or generalise about matters).
3   Avoid mind-reading.
4   Take responsibility for own actions.
5   Avoid monologues, i.e. say what you need to say and then stop.
6   Examine non-verbal communication.

This was to be done tactfully, the therapist approaching the subject by suggesting that each family member might obtain greater satisfaction, and be more likely to achieve their aims without argument, if they examined the way in which they spoke to each other.

Both Mary and her mother appeared interested in this idea. The therapist, therefore, asked each of them to think of a conversation they had had in the past week which had been frustrating to them. They were asked to describe exactly what was said. The therapist then helped them to identify the communication errors which had occurred and then, using role play, modelled a more appropriate response. Following this demonstration they were then asked to try a similar approach but on this occasion, they were to role play themselves. The therapist gave them feedback on their performance (ensuring that some positive feedback was given initially, followed by any constructive criticism plus modelling). At the end of the session, the therapist gave them a sheet of paper with the rules for effective communication written down. They were asked to keep a note of their difficult communications during the week for discussion in the next session but to try, wherever possible, to think of the rules in their conversations.

Further sessions with the family concentrated on their communication. After six such sessions, they appeared to have made great improvements. Ralph's mother, however, complained how tired she was. The therapist commented that this was not surprising considering how much she did for Ralph. Ralph spontaneously expressed a wish that his mother would not do so much. In view of this the therapist suggested a mutual behavioural programme for Ralph and his mother based on the ideas of the 'give to get' principles of behavioural exchange therapy (described in Chapter 8). In other words the therapist explained the principle of mutual reinforcement, and then asked Ralph and his Mother in turn for two changes each they would like to see in the other. The final programme for the first week was as follows:

Ralph
1   To make his own bed every morning.
2   To help mother carry shopping home on Fridays.
Mother
1   To not read Ralph's mail without his permission.
2   To allow Ralph to go out without asking where he is going (Ralph will inform Mother of likely time of return).

After some discussion, both Ralph and his mother agreed to these tasks to be done on a 'give to get' basis.

Thereafter, further sessions were held with an increasing number of reciprocal tasks agreed each week aimed at increasing Ralph's autonomy. This proceeded in a way similar to the case of Calum and Mhairi Dolan in chapter 8.

After seven further sessions, the family seemed happier and more contented. Ralph spent more time away from home enjoying his solitary hobbies. Interactions between Ralph and his mother and sister were much more relaxed and friendly. Arrangements were made for Ralph and his family to have continued access to psychiatric support.

Three years since this programme was introduced, Ralph has only suffered from one minor relapse of his psychotic illness. Although Ralph's case demonstrates that high EE can be important in relapse of schizophrenia, it is important not to assume that all families with a schizophrenic member have high EE. A measuring instrument can be used to assess EE, and further information can be obtained in a book on the subject (Leff & Vaughn, 1985). However, the general principles of education and help with specific problems can be of great benefit to many families with a schizophrenic member.

Summary

·   In many cases the behavioural treatment of the chronic patient aims for care rather than cure.
·   In changing behaviour in the chronic patient there are currently three main groups of techniques:
     1   Operant methods.
     2   Social and task-oriented skills training.
     3   Behavioural family therapy.
·   Negative reinforcement and punishment are rarely used. Response cost, however, may have a role in a behavioural programme.
·   The wishes of the patient and patient's family, as well as the likely outcome of treatment, must always be considered.

· In the use of operant methods, reinforcers may be used which *increase* or *decrease* specified activities.

· Premack's principal states that high-frequency preferred activity can be used to reinforce lower-frequency, non-preferred activity.

· There are many possible pitfalls in the use of operant methods, in particular that of relapse when the programme is discontinued, and the failure of therapy because of the lack of commitment of the whole team.

· In social and task-oriented skills training, coaching, rehearsal and praise are used.

· In behavioural family therapy some of the essential ingredients are education of the family about the illness, and teaching how *expressed emotion* can be altered by various techniques.

11 Treatment of non-phobic anxiety

Anxiety is an almost universal phenomenon. A small amount is often helpful and can improve performance, but as anxiety increases performance is reduced. An inverted U-shaped curve describes this relationship. In pathological anxiety there are usually symptoms of over-activity of the autonomic nervous system: shortness of breath, dizziness, sweating, tremor, palpitations, choking, nausea, depersonalisation or de-realisation, paraesthesia, flushes or chills, chest pain or discomfort, fear of dying or of doing something uncontrolled. In contrast to the anxiety in phobic disorders described in chapter 3, there is no specific object or situation that is feared. Panic attacks can occur out of the blue, with a sudden feeling of fear, terror or apprehension. In the third edition of the *Diagnostic and Statistical Manual of Mental Disorders* by the American Psychiatric Association (1987) *panic disorder* now takes precedence over agoraphobia. Panic disorders are defined as being unexpected as well as not triggered by situations, with at least four of the above symptoms.

A second form of anxiety state is called *generalised anxiety disorder*, and this occurs when the main problem is unrealistic or there is excessive anxiety and worry, which is about various life circumstances, and the focus is not concerned with the anticipation of panic attacks. In panic disorder and generalised anxiety disorder, the problem is that there is no avoided situation, and so treatment has to involve teaching patients new ways of coping with stress. This can be attempted by changing their thoughts or cognitions, clearly an ambitious project, and is known as *cognitive therapy* (Beck & Emery, 1985). There is also a method called **anxiety management training** (Suinn & Richardson, 1971, Meichenbaum 1977, Butler *et al.*, 1987) which focuses on the patient's fears of being unable to cope. These terms describe similar approaches, but as each has a differing emphasis they will be described separately. A large number of patients experience both panic attacks *and* generalised anxiety and the treatment of each requires both types of treatment approach.

Treatment of anxiety is best approached by logically considering:

> Is the patient doing things to bring on anxiety?
> If so the treatment is focused on altering these *precipitating causes*.
> Can the treatment involve changing *behaviour*?
> If so then behavioural treatment is indicated.
> Finally if the above methods fail, then a *cognitive* approach should be tried.

Precipitating causes

Anxiety symptoms are generally caused by either an increased sympathetic outflow, an imbalance between sympathetic and parasympathetic systems or by increased muscular tension. It stands to reason, therefore, that any factors which effect these systems can result in 'anxiety-like' symptoms. Not only can these be misdiagnosed by the medical profession, but they may also be complicated by producing true anxiety symptoms, either by classical conditioning or by the patient's interpretation of the meaning of the symptom.

Some medical conditions which can be confused with anxiety include:

Thyrotoxicosis.
Adrenal tumours.
Carcinoid syndrome.
Zollinger-Ellison syndrome (hypoglycaemia leading to increased sympathetic outflow).
Poorly controlled diabetes.
Paroxysmal atrial tachycardia.

As well as recognised medical syndromes, other physical factors may cause symptoms indistinguishable from anxiety. Examples of these include:

Excessive caffeine intake.
Excessive nicotine.
Excessive alcohol (withdrawal in the form of a 'hangover' is partially characterised by increased sympathetic outflow).
Drug abuse (cannabis excess generally leads to increased vagal output; amphetamines to increased sympathetic output).
Withdrawal from benzodiazepine medication.
Irregular meals leading to hypoglycaemia.
Reactive hypoglycaemia.
Insufficient regular exercise.
Excessive tiredness.

The following case history of a young executive serves to illustrate some of these points.

Case history of man with poor life-style leading to 'anxiety' symptoms

Richard, a 32-year-old unmarried merchant banker, was referred to the clinic with a one year history of severe 'panic episodes'. These episodes could occur at any time of the day or night and consisted of palpitations, sweating and a feeling of impending doom. Each episode lasted for 25–30 minutes and occurred four to six times a day. The patient could not suggest a precipitant for these episodes.

After obtaining the history of presenting complaint, the therapist inquired about Richard's general life-style. It became clear that he woke at 7.00 a.m. and left the house 20 minutes later having had no breakfast. A busy morning at work would also involve him in drinking at least three cups of ground coffee. In addition, Richard smoked approximately 15 cigarettes a day. Lunch consisted of either a sandwich, if he was not too busy, or frequently a bar of chocolate. During the afternoon he would have five to six cups of coffee before finishing work at 6.30 or 7.00 p.m. He would generally then meet friends and eat out in a restaurant, consuming up to a bottle of wine before returning home to bed after midnight. Richard took little exercise and his only hobbies were eating out or visiting the public house to drink. Although he was not overweight, he noticeably lacked tone and had poor posture.

The therapist then explained to Richard that there were multiple factors in his life-style which were probably contributing to his symptoms. Firstly, he had irregular meals which may lead to hypoglycaemia, and this might be added to by his habit of consuming high carbohydrate food on an empty stomach, possibly leading to reactive hypoglycaemia. His smoking habits might also contribute to this, as well as increasing his sympathetic output due to the stimulant effect. His caffeine intake was excessive and, as a stimulant, would increase his sympathetic outflow. The amount of alcohol he was consuming could well contribute to his problem by increasing his symptoms in the morning and also by contributing to morning hypoglycaemia. Finally, he took no exercise although he worked long hours in a sedentary job. His lack of fitness was demonstrated by his resting pulse rate of 98 beats per minute.

Clearly no-one could expect Richard to revolutionise his entire life style immediately. The therapist, therefore, asked him what he would feel able to tackle initially. Richard was sceptical that his life-style had any effect on his symptoms at all but eventually agreed to test this out. He agreed to eat three meals a day of the following foods:

Breakfast – Bowl of cornflakes and milk
Lunch   – One round of sandwiches (meat, fish or cheese)
Dinner   – In restaurant

In addition he agreed to stop drinking ground coffee, and to change to the decaffeinated variety. The therapist warned Richard that when many people stopped or reduced their caffeine intake, they would suffer from withdrawal symptoms. These usually consisted of a headache, which generally started 24 to 48 hours after the reduction in caffeine, and could be accompanied by sweating and tremulousness. These symptoms should reduce after approximately 24 hours and were evidence of caffeine dependence. Richard was asked to record his success with these changes and to record the time and situation of any 'panic' episodes.

At the end of a week, Richard reported that he was felling much better than before. He had experienced a mild headache after reducing his intake of fresh coffee, but this had settled quickly. Nearly all his 'funny turns' were happening in the morning, and he felt that he would like to reduce his alcohol intake to below the recommended limit of 21 units. A full drinking history was taken from Richard, and the therapist advised ways in which he could pace and slow his drinking, as well as advising him on low alcohol and alcohol-free beverages. Richard felt that he could reduce his alcohol intake best by travelling to the restaurant or public house in his car as he would never drink and drive. He could do this by refusing lifts from others and volunteering to take others in his car (over the past few years, he felt that he 'owed' most of his friends a large number of car journeys).

When Richard returned two weeks later, he had been remarkably successful in reducing his alcohol intake and did not require any of the specific intervention for reducing excessive alcohol described in chapter 6. The therapist praised him for his rapid and excellent progress. He was only complaining of 'funny turns' once or twice a week. Richard was then asked if he wished to concentrate on consolidating his gains for a while or to start to introduce another behavioural change. He felt that he did not wish to reduce his smoking at this time, but enquired about exercise. It was explained to him that it was extremely important for him to find a form of exercise that he could enjoy and perform regularly and not something which would be a penance. Regular exercise would not only increase his general fitness and reduce his heart rate and tendency to palpitations, but would also give him another interest apart from work. Indeed, regular aerobic exercise has been shown to have a beneficial effect on people with true anxiety symptoms (Morgan & Goldston, 1987).

Richard felt that he would hate jogging or running. After some discussion with the therapist, it became clear that while at school, Richard had been a member of the school swimming team. He had not swum for several years and had not thought about restarting as he realised that at his age he was too old to take part in true competitive swimming. The therapist suggested that he might like to think of other alternatives and should visit the local baths and find out about life-saving classes, long-distance swimming clubs and clubs for adults. Richard agreed to this and agreed to the goal of going swimming at least three times a week.

Over the next few weeks, Richard became increasingly enthusiastic about his rediscovered hobby of swimming. He had joined a club for people over 30 which met twice a week and organised galas with races for different age groups. He had also managed to reduce his smoking and was planning to stop as he felt it had a deleterious effect on his swimming performance. The incidence of 'panic' episodes was now negligible, and this improvement was maintained at one year follow-up.

Behavioural treatments

These include

Avoiding avoidance
Prediction testing
Voluntary hyperventilation
Pacing tapes
Relaxation training

Avoiding avoidance

There may seem a contradiction here as in anxiety disorders by definition there is no avoidance. However, there often is subtle avoidance, for example avoidance of activities that might bring on symptoms, or the use of avoidance strategies to relieve symptoms which have already started. As an example of the former can be given the case of a 54-year-old man who had made a good recovery from a heart attack, but avoided sexual intercourse with his wife, because his initial symptoms began when having intercourse, and he feared bringing on another attack. Treatment involved him facing up to the feared activity, and when he had done so he made a rapid recovery.

The use of subtle avoidance strategies to relieve symptoms can demand considerable therapeutic skills. A patient may conceal how disabled they are by anxiety and make seemingly plausible excuses, for example 'I really prefer to work at home, and think of all the money I save in train fares' – this from a patient who turned out to have actual phobic avoidance of going out of her house. Similarly, another patient made tiny tapping movements of her fingers to relieve anxiety and this was challenged by her therapist in a session. It then turned out that these movements were done to 'ward off harm' and after this other features of obsessive-compulsive disorder were revealed. The treatment of obsessive-compulsive disorder is described in chapter 4, but this case is mentioned here as an example of subtle avoidance.

Prediction testing

This is a technique based on the idea that if the patient can be encouraged to devise an experiment to test out what in fact will happen if certain experiences are undergone then it will not be as bad in reality as he had feared. It differs from subtle avoidance as there is no avoidance, however subtle, and a purely artificial situation has to be worked out to carry out a behavioural experiment.

John was a young man with general anxiety symptoms which were especially bad if he thought people were looking at him. He never avoided any social situations, but he was asked to devise an imagined situation that would bring on the most symptoms, and he pointed out that if he was to walk past a group of school-children he would feel very bad indeed, because this would make him very self conscious. He would fear that the children might laugh at him, and then he would become awkward and make a fool of himself. He had no children of his own and in the normal way would never come into contact with children. After some discussion he agreed that it would be useful to walk past a school just as the children were coming out and force himself to do this difficult task on a number of occasions. Prediction testing in this way served to prove to him that the worst feared consequences would not happen, and was a useful part of the therapeutic strategy in his case.

Voluntary hyperventilation

This technique has a long history in behavioural treatments, and inhalation of a gas consisting of 65% carbon dioxide and 35% oxygen was advocated by Wolpe in 1958. However, Wolpe suggests that the effect is not a direct pharmacological one, but symptoms are induced such as shortness of breath, flushing, paraesthesia and dizziness. Nowadays similar symptoms are induced by voluntary hyperventilation alone, and the aim is to enable exposure to these symptoms so that habituation can occur. Instructions to the patient are given along these lines:

Many of the symptoms you feel might be due to the fact that you breath too fast. When you do this it has the effect of reducing the concentration of carbon dioxide in your blood. When the carbon dioxide gets below a certain critical level it effects nerve conduction in the body so that you get the alteration in sensation we call pins and needles (or paraesthesia in medical jargon) along with other unpleasant symptoms you associate with anxiety. By *deliberately* over-breathing now we can do the experiment of seeing if this happens in the safe situation of this clinic.

After about two minutes of hard over-breathing the patient is asked to report what *actual* symptoms were experienced, and then asked whether these feelings are similar to those experienced in a panic attack. Most patients have difficulty in performing over-breathing to a sufficient extent to reproduce symptoms if just asked to do so. For this reason it is better for the therapist to perform the exercise along with the patient. The resultant symptoms and signs produced in the therapist can be an additional useful learning experience for the patient. Any therapist should remember that this technique does produce a number of unpleasant symptoms and it is advisable for the therapist not to drive for at least 30 minutes after performing this exercise. Getting the patient to over-breathe is useful in two ways: it helps put symptoms in perspective – 'Well, I survived that perhaps that real thing is not going to kill me after all', and also by providing practice in exposure to feared symptoms and their consequences.

There are some medical conditions where hard hyperventilation may be contraindicated, for example recent myocardial infarction, and some forms of obstructive airways disease. In these cases the therapist may demonstrate the effect of voluntary hyperventilation on himself/herself and then tell the patient what effect it had. It is also sound practice to use modelling in this way with any patient reluctant to use this technique.

Pacing tapes

Voluntary hyperventilation may be useful in many patients with panic attacks but there may be some difficulty enabling the technique to be practised outside the clinic situation. Clark *et al.* (1985) have devised a way round this by using audio-tape recordings of a voice saying 'breathe in' followed by a two second pause then 'breath out' followed by a two second pause, to be repeated in this fashion over a 10-minute period. The therapist chooses the rate most suitable for the patient, and patients are asked to follow the pacing on the tape. Next the patient is asked to turn the tape off and carry on breathing at the same pace for progressively longer periods. They are then given practice in controlled breathing to reduce the sensations that occur in panic.

Relaxation training

Relaxation can be seen as a coping skill, that once acquired can be used by the patient to reduce symptoms in anxiety disorders. It is something positive a patient can do in an anxiety attack and serves to reduce the sense of helplessness. In some oriental cultures relaxation is part of the life-style, but not so in most Western cultures. Therefore relaxation has to be *taught* and it is worth emphasising to patients that, as with other things that have to be taught, a number of practice sessions will be needed. Various methods are available (see Bernstein & Borkovec, 1973), but rather than stick rigidly to any one of the published procedures the authors have devised their own which is reproduced in Appendix 1. It is our practice to go through the technique with the patient and make a tape recording of this. In this way the details can be tailor made to the individual patient, and the tape can be given to the patient for home practice. As a further refinement, tapes could be played through a personal stereo, so that the actual instructions would be heard at the appropriate time and place.

It is wise to remember that relaxation has only a very limited role in helping to treat anxiety and should rarely, if ever, be used alone. For example, most people can be taught to relax at home. However, if after being taught relaxation, the person is taken for the first time into a light aircraft and told to jump with a parachute, they are likely to experience anxiety. Any amount of relaxation training will not change this in most cases. Thus although relaxation may be helpful for general stress and tension, it is not helpful for situational anxiety.

Cognitive treatments

These include

> Anxiety management training
> Beck's cognitive treatment

Anxiety management training

There are four stages:

1 Explanation to the patient for the symptoms.
2 Teaching how to face up to the symptoms.
3 Teaching coping with the feeling of being overwhelmed.
4 Reinforcing self-statements.

These stages in treatment will be illustrated first by the case of James who was an extremely anxious 55-year-old man, who had a large number of complaints. He became breathless for no apparent reason, had sensations of 'pins and needles' in both arms, and a feeling of discomfort in his abdomen, which he described as 'like butterflies in the tummy'. He experienced these symptoms for no reason that could be discovered and his doctor could not find any organic cause for them. The symptoms had started about a year before and the only significant factor that emerged from exhaustive interviews was that his brother who was two years his senior, had suffered a heart attack at the time James began to have symptoms, but his brother had now made a complete recovery.

Explanation for the symptoms

A session was spent allowing James to talk about the symptoms, and helping him give him an explanation for them. It was pointed out that when he becomes anxious he breathes too fast, and it was explained that this lowers the carbon dioxide levels in his blood too much and is the cause of the 'pins and needles'.

Similarly, he was given an explanation for the abdominal discomfort:

> When you feel tense you become aware of sensations from your gut contractions that you would not otherwise experience – it is a normal physiological happening that you are pathologically aware of due to your over arousal.

Learning how to face up to the symptoms

James had to learn that breathing fast was a symptom of anxiety. He could accept the explanation given above at an intellectual level but this alone did not seem to help:

'I believe what you say but this does not change the way I feel.' The key to teaching him to face up to the symptoms was to encourage repeated coping self-statements, and these were written onto a card which he carried around with him all the time. James's card looked like this:

1   Breathing too fast is something I do when I get anxious.
2   Breathing too fast removes the carbon dioxide from my blood and then I get the pins and needles.
3   Butterflies in my tummy are due to anxiety.
4   If I just calm down and wait, these anxiety symptoms will go away.

Each of these statements was arrived at after some discussion between James and his therapist, and each one was only written on the card after he had agreed that it was a meaningful statement that was *relevant* to his difficulty. He was given the homework task of reading the card each evening and carrying it around in his pocket. Whenever he experienced a symptom he was to pull out his card and read it to himself.

This approach was helpful most of the time, but special techniques were needed at times when he became overwhelmed with a symptom.

Coping with the feeling of being overwhelmed

At times utter panic would cause James to tremble such that he could not even hold the card still enough to read it. To deal with these attacks he was taught systematic muscular relaxation exercises (see Appendix 1 for details), which he carried out once with the therapist giving the instructions, but on the second occasion the session was tape-recorded and he had the homework task of playing the tape at home to perfect the technique. This turned out to be enough to terminate 9 out of 10 panic attacks, but he still had rare occasions when the anxiety was overwhelming. To combat the severest attacks he carried a portable tape-recorder with the relaxation instructions, and this was usually effective. We do not know if this partial success was because the familiar voice of his therapist was reassuring, or because of some other mechanism.

Reinforcing self-statements

The main aim of anxiety management training is to give the patient himself the skills to cope with anxiety, so that he is soon able to relieve symptoms without the therapist having to intervene. In order to give him this independence it is useful for the patient to give the reinforcement for success, taking over this role that the therapist initially has. In practice the therapist praised James for success, for example:

> You reduced your rate of breathing very well last session, that's excellent.

James himself later on gave himself praise where this was due:

> When I read my card, took a deep breath, and waited a while, the panic went away: I'm managing much better now.

One such self-reinforcing statement that James invented could be used by the many patients who use this technique:

Nothing succeeds like success!

Beck's cognitive therapy

The model here is: that it is not events themselves but people's expectations and interpretation of events which causes anxiety. Individuals overestimate the danger in a situation and start responding in a way that was originally meant to protect us from harm, for example flight or fight.

Within Beck's model two levels of disturbed thinking have been described:

1   Automatic thoughts.
2   Thinking errors.

Clark (1988) has further refined the cognitive model of panic, stating that individuals experience panic attacks because of a tendency to interpret a range of bodily sensations in a catastrophic fashion. This interpretation leads to a further increase in bodily sensations and a vicious circle ensues. Salkovskis & Clark (1990) in an experiment using volunteer subjects, showed that hyperventilation played an important role in panic attacks *only* if the effect of the hyperventilation was interpreted by the subject in a catastrophic way.

Once the vicious circle is established two further factors make the situation worse. Firstly, hyper-vigilance makes the patient repeatedly scan their body, and so more symptoms are noticed. Secondly, the avoidance of certain activities maintains the negative ideas, for example the idea that exercise will bring on a heart attack can lead to avoidance of exercise, leading to the patient never testing himself out in a situation where exercise is necessary.

The principles of cognitive treatment for anxiety are similar to those of cognitive therapy for depression described in chapter 12. The principle of treating negative thoughts by examination of the evidence is the same, as well as the use of highly structured sessions and homework assignments.

Teaching control of 'automatic thoughts'

Douglas, a 22-year-old man had suffered from panic attacks since childhood. In an attack he felt:

. . . unreal, as if I'm not really here, I think I am going to swallow my tongue, although I realise this is a silly idea, and then I will lose control of myself.

The panic attacks had worsened about three months ago for no apparent reason. The symptoms prevented his full enjoyment of life, as he lived in dread of an attack coming on, but despite this they did not unduly interfere with his job as a bricklayer. He lived at home with his parents and had a reasonable social life. He had recognised that alcohol brought about short term symptom relief, and was developing a reliance on beer that threatened to become a serious problem. It was explained to Douglas that he had to learn how to face up to his symptoms rather than use alcohol.

The symptom of depersonalisation, in which he felt unreal, was one of the most distressing to him as he believed it was a symptom of serious physical illness which might cause him to die. He was given the self-help book to read entitled *Living with Fear* (Marks, 1978) and gained considerably from reading about another patient with depersonalisation. This was used as the starting point for cognitive therapy:

THERAPIST: So you now realise you are not the only one with this symptom. Can we now look at the evidence for this idea of yours that you are not really here, not flesh and blood?

PATIENT: I feel odd, sort of freaked out, as if my arms and legs do not belong to me.

THERAPIST: So the idea that your arms and legs do not belong to you leads to anxiety?

PATIENT: Yes

THERAPIST: And what happens eventually?

PATIENT: The attack passes, and normal feelings return to my arms and legs.

THERAPIST: What does that experience suggest to you?

PATIENT: That the attack will pass and is not dangerous.

THERAPIST: So the attack is short-lived and not lethal. What do you feel is the cause of it?

PATIENT: Well, since reading that book, I think it is just a horrible form of anxiety attack.

THERAPIST: So, would you say that rather than believing these episodes to be evidence of serious illness, an alternative explanation could be that in an anxiety attack, the symptom of losing sensation in your limbs leads to further anxiety, but without good reason as eventually the attack passes?

PATIENT: I suppose you are right.

THERAPIST: How could you test this theory out?

PATIENT: Well, I also get really anxious if I go to a party. I usually drink before I go or I won't go at all. If I go to the party on Saturday and not drink I could try and see whether I have any experiences which are similar to those that I have during an attack.

Douglas was able to do this and convinced himself that his feelings of depersonalisation were symptoms of anxiety which were unpleasant but temporary, and therefore did not cause any long-term damage.

At the next session, the therapist started to help Douglas to look at his belief that he might swallow his tongue during an attack.

THERAPIST: Can we examine this belief that you may swallow your tongue. Firstly let us see what is the evidence for this belief.

Table 11.1. *Self-coping cue card: first example*

Symptom	Self-statement
My arms and legs do not belong to me	This is an anxiety symptom which I know from experience will pass
I feel I might swallow my tongue	I never have swallowed my tongue, and I know I can't. This is due to focusing too much attention on my throat, which is due to dry mouth, which in turn is an anxiety symptom

PATIENT: Well, I feel as if I'm going to.

THERAPIST: Any other evidence?

PATIENT: No.

THERAPIST: Shall we look at the evidence against this belief, then?

PATIENT: I have never heard of anyone swallowing their tongue, and although I have had this experience hundreds of times, I have not swallowed it so far.

THERAPIST: That's fine but what could be causing it then?

PATIENT: Could it be a symptom of anxiety, my mouth does feel dry?

THERAPIST: That is likely, as in anxiety the autonomic nervous system is overactive, and the parasympathetic part of the autonomic nervous system controls secretion of saliva. This would make your mouth feel dry, and may well make you feel as if your are swallowing your tongue.

PATIENT: That is alright as far as it goes, but I still do not see how focusing attention on my throat brings on the symptom

THERAPIST: How could we test that out?

PATIENT: I could try to think very hard now about my tongue and see what happens.

THERAPIST: Let's try that as we are sitting here. Just think about your tongue for a few minutes . . .

PATIENT: I see what you mean, I am now aware of sensations I did not have a few minutes ago.

THERAPIST: Exactly. So now you can see how attention to your throat has brought about the symptom.

The patient was also asked to write down on cue cards the rational response to each symptom. Cue cards, originally devised by Meichenbaum, can in practice be incorporated into Beck's cognitive therapy. This patient ended up with these cards which he found useful to carry about, and one of these cards is illustrated in Table 11.1.

These *rational responses* had been worked out by the patient as he filled in his *thought diaries*. In a thought diary the patient is asked to write down the negative automatic thought, the evidence for and against each thought and the rational response to the thought. In the early stages of therapy, it is often useful to include a space for recording the external circumstances at the time the thought occurred as well as the resultant emotion from the thought, so that the patient can recognise how thoughts affect emotions. Towards the end of therapy, it is useful to record the underlying assumption as well as the negative automatic thoughts so that these can be challenged. As there will be fewer underlying assumptions than all the varieties of negative automatic thought that an individual may have, then this is a way of getting to the grassroots of the thinking errors.

Gillian is a 24-year-old secretary who begins to have anxiety symptoms each day before setting off for work. She dreads going to work on the underground train, and begins to sweat, has pains in her stomach, feels sick, and fears she will pass out. When she enters the train she feels all these symptoms become worse and in addition she experiences palpitations. Despite having these symptoms since the age of 18 years when she started work, she has *never* avoided work nor has she avoided travel on the underground train.

The very first attack of anxiety that Gillian remembered was in school assembly when she was 17 years of age. At that time she feared that she would pass out, and experienced palpitations. After this episode she had been allowed to avoid school assembly whenever she felt anxious. This had happened on numerous occasions.

The *behavioural formulation* was that learnt avoidance of a feared situation (crowded school assembly) had generalised to the crowded underground train. She had never had to face the school assembly when younger, and that particular situation was no longer relevant to her life. At the present time, she was regularly facing a feared situation, but as is sometimes the case, the anxiety would not habituate despite regular and long exposure.

When standing at the train platform she had a bad attack of anxiety, and she said to herself:

This is it. This train will never come. I am going to freak out and collapse. I am breathing too fast and my heart is going too fast. I must give up my job and stop putting myself through this torture every day.

She was then asked to record these thoughts each day on a chart, and in the next session the therapist examined the *evidence* for each thought with her:

THERAPIST: So what makes you think you will freak out and die?
PATIENT: I feel this pounding in my chest. It is most unpleasant, and then I feel I am going to die.
THERAPIST: What is the evidence that you will collapse in an attack?
PATIENT: Well there is not any so far, but there is always a first time!
THERAPIST: So the pounding in your chest leads to the thought that you might die, even though you think this is unlikely. If we could think of a way to bring on the attack just by exercise, then perhaps you could see that the extra activity of your heart is a way of your heart providing more blood needed for exercise.
PATIENT: That is an idea, how could I do that?

THERAPIST: If you were to run up and down on the spot now then see if it produces similar symptoms, that could prove something to you.

The patient agreed to do this activity for about three minutes, and the therapist did it at the same time, they then each measured the others pulse rate.

THERAPIST: Right, so how do you feel now and what does that tell you?
PATIENT: My heart is pounding in the same way that I worry about. Your pulse is even more rapid than mine after the exercise, and yet you look fine. So I suppose that I must conclude that exercise brings on the same symptoms, and I accept this in this situation. I suppose that a possible explanation for my symptoms is that I overreact to my normal bodily functioning.

The awareness of her breathing and heart beating were explained to her in terms of over arousal of the autonomic nervous system. This over arousal had led her to conclude (erroneously) that she would collapse or go mad.

Later in treatment she made cue cards based on her thought diaries, and these are shown in Table 11.2.

With the regular use of these cue cards Gillian felt somewhat less anxious about going to work, but on a 0 to 8 scale of symptom severity, where 0 indicated no anxiety and 8 indicated the worst possible symptomatology, she scored 8 at the start and 6 at the end of six sessions with no indication that anxiety would decrease further. She had previously been treated with a variety of tablets to reduce anxiety with no effect. It is unusual, but not unknown for patients to have anxiety without avoidance, as in this case. Gillian was praised for continually facing the feared situation, and the dangers of not doing so were pointed out to her. Learning to *live with fear* is a necessity for some patients, although they can be reassured that as the years go by the intensity of fear does diminish.

Thinking errors
Some of the main thinking errors in anxiety disorders can be categorised as:

Table 11.2. *Self-coping cue card: second example*

Symptom	Self-statement
This sweating is unbearable	The sweats mean I'm anxious, nothing more
I think I'm going to pass out	I never have passed out and it's not likely now
Palpitations are terrible	Palpitations are just anxiety symptoms, you won't die

> exaggerating
> catastrophising
> overgeneralising

Illustration of 'exaggerating'

Walter sat in his hospital bed recovering from his operation. He was 'terrified of everything' but before his operation had been a successful garage owner with no particular anxieties. He was 65 years old and making a good recovery from a pneumonectomy operation for lung cancer which was surgically very successful. His wife had recovered from a breast cancer operation five years before and was now completely well, but he knew she had been through a great deal of pain and he dreaded going through similar suffering. On the day that he was first seen he was waiting to have a liver scan to check on whether the cancer involved his liver. He was very preoccupied with pain and anxiety and said:

I will never be able to survive all this pain

THERAPIST: makes you think that?

PATIENT: No one can control the pain – there is nothing I can do, nothing the doctors can do.

THERAPIST: What is the evidence for that.

PATIENT: When I had the last pain-killer injection the effect wore off after two hours.

THERAPIST: What happened then?

PATIENT: Two hours after that they gave me some more, but they can't go on doing this for ever can they?

THERAPIST: Are you getting the same amount of medication now as after the operation?

PATIENT: No they are gradually reducing it.

THERAPIST: What could be the reason for this?

PATIENT: The pain *is* getting less. If I have survived so far, perhaps I can survive longer.

Illustration of catastrophising

WALTER: I've not had a night's sleep since the operation, without proper sleep I'll die.

THERAPIST: First of all are you sure that it is true that you have not slept since the operation?

PATIENT: Well, the nurses say I have slept, but I feel as if I have not.

THERAPIST: So could you could be overestimating the lack of sleep?

PATIENT: I suppose I have to believe the nurses, but the important thing to me is how I feel. I feel terrible just as if I have had no sleep.

THERAPIST: You also said that you thought you might die through lack of sleep. What is the evidence for that?

PATIENT: I feel as if I have not slept, and I feel like death!

THERAPIST: So you mean you feel terrible, and conclude you are going to die. Is there any other explanation?

PATIENT: I could feel terrible for any number of reasons . . . I have just had a major operation . . . I am getting all this medication.

THERAPIST: Yes it sounds as if you have inflated the importance of lack of sleep. People can survive perfectly well with less sleep than they think they need. As the pain dies down, and when you leave hospital you will start to lead a more normal routine, and sleep patterns will probably become more normal.

PATIENT: I shall tell myself no one died through lack of sleep.

Illustration of overgeneralisation

PATIENT: My wife was in terrible pain, I know I could not cope with that. People with cancer die a slow, painful death.

THERAPIST: Can you tell me what this idea of yours is based upon?

PATIENT: My friend at work had stomach trouble for a long time. He had a great deal of pain, and then they found out that he had cancer, and after a lot of suffering he died.

THERAPIST: Alright, that is one example of cancer causing a lingering painful condition. But what about your wife's cancer?

PATIENT: She was in great pain.

THERAPIST: But how long did it last, and what was the outcome?

PATIENT: Three weeks after the operation her pain went, and now they say she has made a complete recovery.

THERAPIST: What can you conclude from this?

PATIENT: There are different outcomes for different people?

THERAPIST: Yes, and what about the significance of the pain?

PATIENT: I suppose it does not necessarily mean that the outcome will be bad. Perhaps it depends on other things like the kind of cancer, and what stage it has reached by the time the doctors treat it.

The use of imagery techniques

The final case in this chapter is very unusual, as it is an example of one of those rare cases in which meaning was essential to the patient's understanding of the symptoms. Usually it is not necessary to go to such lengths, but in this case the simpler methods had failed.

A 25-year-old married woman had difficulty eating in public. She had completed all the exposure therapy exercises to her avoided situations, similar to those described in chapter 3, but despite overcoming avoidance, still felt very anxious whenever she had to eat anything when someone was looking at her.

THERAPIST: Sometimes people have an image in their mind which leads them to become anxious in a situation. If we can run through this image rather like playing back a film in your mind it could help. Please close your eyes, and imagine you are sitting at a table with a plate of food in front of you, how does that make you feel?

PATIENT: I feel anxious. It is a horrible feeling, my stomach is contracting and waves of panic pass over me.

THERAPIST: Now, you have told me that you have had this symptom since childhood. Can you try to recall when it first started and how you felt at that time.

PATIENT: (after a few minutes silence): I was a child at school. We were having school dinners, and I can remember this dinner lady standing over me. She insisted that I finished all the food on my plate, and this made me very anxious because I knew I could not.

THERAPIST: Now tell me what is happening, and what you are feeling.

PATIENT: I am now angry with that dinner lady.

THERAPIST: Why do you think you are angry?

PATIENT: I am sure it is because of her that I have problems now, but I can't get back at her now after all these years . . . she may not even be alive.

THERAPIST: You are right, you cannot get back at her. However, we have an idea here that your pent up anger might still be causing you problems. Can we test this out in some way?

PATIENT: Get the anger out you mean . . . then if I feel better it may have proved something?

THERAPIST: Yes and one way to do this is to imagine this dinner lady is really sitting here with us in this room, and you give her a piece of your mind. Could you try that now?

PATIENT: You bossy power-crazed bitch, why don't you pick on someone your own size instead of pushing little children around . . . you in your position of authority ought to understand how difficult it is for children to eat in a hurry . . . they only have small stomachs you know, and if you make a child anxious it makes it even worse . . . If I could get hold of you I would teach you a lesson you won't forget . . .

The homework exercise was to write an essay entitled 'Instructions to Dinner Ladies', in which she was encouraged to put her feelings onto paper, as a way of further playing out the imagery and re-living the emotional experience. Further sessions were spent reviewing the homework, and encouraging expression of anger. The use of imagery here produced a good result in a case where exposure *in vivo* alone was unsatisfactory, and the patient remained symptom-free at one year follow-up.

Summary

·   Non-phobic anxiety can be divided into panic disorder and generalised anxiety disorder.

·   If there are precipitating causes for anxiety such as overindulgence in coffee, and the inability to change an impossible life-style, and these should be dealt with first, by such techniques as information giving and activity scheduling.

·   Next, behavioural therapy involves avoidance of subtle avoidance, prediction testing, voluntary hyperventilation, the use of pacing tapes and relaxation training.

·   A coping model of treatment has been described by Meichenbaum.

·   Beck's model of anxiety leads to treatment of negative automatic thoughts, and the correction of logical errors such as exaggeration, catastrophisation, and overgeneralisation.

·   Other specifically cognitive techniques can involve the use of imagery, but are rarely needed in practice.

12 *Treatment of depression*

The experience of depression is so common as to be almost part of the human condition, and this makes it easy to empathise with depressed patients. However, it is not just sadness that requires treatment but when sadness becomes severe it merges into depression. Some classification is needed to decide which cases of depression require treatment: the *Diagnostic and Statistical Manual of Mental Disorders* classification divides mood disorders into bipolar disorders and depressive disorders. The essential feature of depressive disorders is one or more periods of depression *without* a history of either manic or hypomanic episodes. There are two depressive disorders: major depression, in which there is one or more major depressive episodes; and dysthymia, in which there is a history of depressed mood more days than not for at least two years and in which, during the first two years of the disturbance, the condition did not meet the criterion for a major depressive episode. It is in dysthymia, which was formerly known as *neurotic depression*, where cognitive and behavioural approaches are commonly used. In this condition as well as periods of depressed mood, there is usually: poor appetite or overeating, sleep difficulties, low energy, low self esteem, poor concentration or difficulty making decisions, and feelings of hopelessness.

In the assessment of the suitability for treatment the severity of depression is important. The most severe cases may require organic treatments such as medication or electroconvulsive therapy (ECT) as well as a period in hospital, and a combination of cognitive and organic therapy is often used. It is useful to measure severity of depression with a rating scale such as the Beck Depression Inventory (BDI; Beck, 1978). This is a 21-item self rating scale which allows assessment of overall depressive symptoms. Those scoring less than 10 are not depressed, 10 to 19 are mildly depressed, 20 to 25 are moderately depressed and above 26 indicates severe depression. There is also a 13-item BDI (shortened version) which allows for quick assessment of depression (Beck *et al.*, 1974). Another factor in the assessment of suitability is whether the cognitive approach appeals to a particular patient: the way to discover this is to describe what cognitive therapy involves and recommend a self-help manual with a cognitive bias, for example *Coping with Depression* by I. Blackburn. The patient is then likely to report back at the next session whether or not this is the approach for them.

A variety of cognitive and behavioural techniques have been advocated in the treatment of depression. This has come about partially because of a dissatisfaction with the traditional psychotherapies, and also a growing realisation that medication alone will probably never provide the solution to a complex multifactorial condition such as depression. Cognitive and behavioural therapy for depression has made a great impact in the last decade largely due to the work of Lewinsohn (1975), Beck *et al.* (1979), Seligman (1975) and Weissman & Paykel (1974).

These treatments consist of techniques aimed mainly at changing *behaviour* on the one hand, and those aimed at changing *cognitions* on the other. This is an artificial distinction however, as behaviour and cognitions interact with each other and with other factors as shown in Fig. 12.1. Despite this distinction, it is useful to describe *behavioural* treatments separately from *cognitive* ones.

One of the early advocates of *behavioural* treatments was Lewinsohn who has suggested four categories of intervention:

1   Techniques aimed at increasing activity.
2   Techniques aimed at reducing unwanted behaviour.
3   Techniques aimed at increasing pleasure.
4   Techniques aimed at enhancing skills.

Lewinsohn's approach will be illustrated by the treatment of Mary a 45-year-old housewife with two teenage children, who had become depressed in the last two years. She herself said 'The children no longer need me like they did, and I have lost all interest in my former hobbies, that was all such a long time ago. I am a very boring person. I just want to sit around the house all day. I know I eat too much, I just can't stop myself. I feel very unattractive, none of my clothes fit me and I can't be bothered to buy any new ones'.

Mary sat around the house all day unable to do anything constructive, and so the initial target was *increase the patient's activity level*. It was decided to use *social reinforcement* to start the process and various activities were discussed with Mary. She finally agreed that she could do something quite simple such as make a telephone call which was reinforced by attention and interest from the therapist. Next she agreed to write a letter, but at the next session had failed to complete the task saying 'I just couldn't think of what to say'. In the session it was agreed she could simply write a short note to her therapist saying 'This is from me, signed Mary', as long as she wrote it and posted it herself. This was the beginning of a series of tasks, of increasing complexity which Mary was gradually able to accomplish. The point to note here is that Mary had said that she could not do anything at all: getting her to write a one line note herself was a way to begin treatment.

The next phase was to *reduce unwanted behaviour*. Mary spent a great deal of her time thinking about the negative aspects of her life 'I'm a

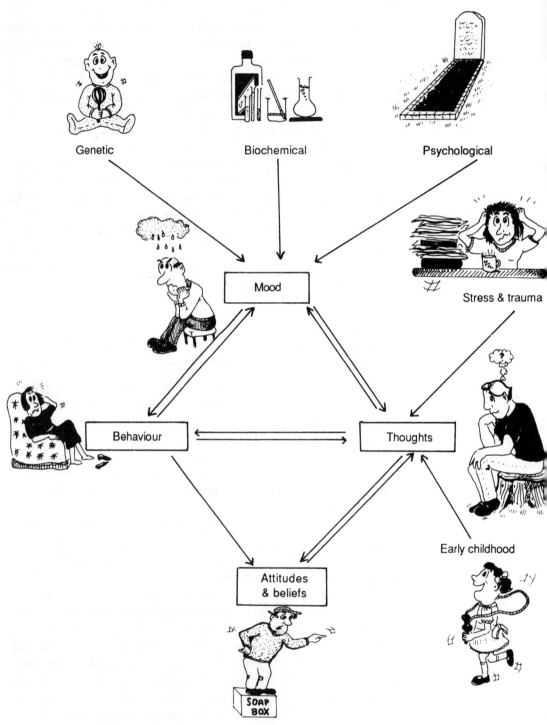

useless, unattractive person who can't do anything'. She was given a
course of *thought stopping* directed at these negative thoughts (this
technique is described in chapter 4). She was also given the behavioural
treatment for obesity as described in chapter 6.

Fig. 12.1. A model of
depression.

After this, sessions were directed at increasing *the amount of pleasurable activity in her life*. Lewinsohn & Graf (1973) described a number of activities that tended to be mood elevating: being relaxed, thinking about something good in the future, having peace and quiet. Achieving all of these appealed to Mary, but she said 'I feel tense all the time, I just have no idea of how to relax'. She was given a course of *relaxation therapy* (see Appendix 1 for details) to help with this. While relaxed she was asked to imagine herself at her favourite holiday resort.

Finally the target became *enhancing skills*. On discussing various possibilities with Mary it was discovered that she used to be a keen amateur artist, and was skilled in drawing and painting. But now she said 'I couldn't even draw a straight line'. At the next session she was given a pencil and some paper and asked to draw a line not bothering about whether it was straight or not. She achieved this, and was given the homework task of drawing three lines on a sheet of paper as straight as she could. By gradually increasing the difficulty of the tasks in this way Mary gradually acquired the confidence to paint in watercolours again.

These four techniques had taken up eight treatment sessions. Several important goals had been achieved, and the Beck Depression Score was reduced from 26 to 19, but there was room for further progress especially in the area of her negative thoughts. This emphasises the message from Fig. 12.1: behaviour and cognitions are intimately linked, and so therapy has to involve both components. Mary's subsequent therapy moved towards more cognitive approaches, but the use of these methods are described further, using other cases.

Increasing the amount of *pleasure* patients can experience is at the core of the Lewinsohn's behavioural therapy of depression; so this will be described in detail using a different case:

Learning mastery and pleasure

The theory behind 'mastery and pleasure' states that a person needs positive reinforcers to feel good about himself, and the individual is 'stroked' by the environment if something pleasing happens, for example someone pays him a compliment, and is also made to feel good by achieving control over the environment in some way. The term *mastery* is used by Lewinsohn and Beck to mean a sense of accomplishment when performing a specific task. *Pleasure* means the pleasant, enjoyable feelings associated with a specific activity. Mastery and pleasure are rated on a 10-point scale where 0 = zero mastery (pleasure) experienced, and 10 = maximum mastery experienced.

Anne was brought for therapy by her husband who said she had become totally unlike her usual self. She was a 44-year-old housewife with two grown up children and said:

I just don't feel like a genuine person any more. I can't seem to feel much at all. It's as if I'm not really here.

The therapist's first objective was to find out why Anne did not engage in any pleasurable activities, and when this was put to Anne she replied:

I do not deserve to have fun. Nothing means anything to me.

At this point therapy could have focused either on these negative cognitions (cognitive therapy), or on increasing the fun in her life by activity level changes (behavioural). The behavioural approach of increasing mastery and pleasure was used, because the history suggested a lack of pleasurable activities that might be easier to modify than the cognitions.

Anne completed the following **activity schedule**:

Monday	*M*	*P*
7–8 a.m. got up, dressed, breakfast	0	0
8–10 a.m. sat in chair with newspaper	0	0
11–12 noon dozed off	0	1
12–1 p.m. lunch	0	0
1–3 p.m. sat in front of TV	0	1

This showed that all activities gave Anne little pleasure, and no sense of mastery. She had been asked to rate her activities for the whole day but given up at 3.00 p.m. saying that there was no point in it. She said that she could never concentrate enough to take what she read in the newspaper. She was given the homework task of reading one page only each day. She was to tell her husband about this each evening when he returned from work.

She doubted whether she could complete this task and failed on the first day. However, her husband picked a very short article for her to read the next day and she was able to complete this with his encouragement. The therapist then tried to find other activities for Anne to tackle, and it was discovered that she used to be a keen swimmer:

ANNE: But the thought of going to a swimming pool fills me with dread.
THERAPIST: What is the first thought you get if I ask you to plan a trip to the pool?
ANNE: I have not got a swimming costume!

It is quite typical for depressed patients to react in this way. Seemingly small difficulties become unsurpassable, and this was dealt with adopting a behaviourial strategy to help her overcome a practical problem:

Anne was given the homework task of buying a swimming costume in the first place, followed by going to the swimming pool. Howeve,r a serious problem then arose: Anne flatly refused to carry out this task. She was therefore given a series of sessions of **graduated exposure** along the lines described for phobic patients in chapter 3.

After this she was able to take her first swim for many years. Using a similar approach Anne was also able to increase her pleasure and mastery of other activities such as going shopping. At the end of a total of 12 sessions her ratings for mastery and pleasure were significantly improved, as was her depression score. At follow-up six months later these scores for a typical day were:

	M	P
7–8 a.m got up, dressed, breakfast	3	4
8–10 a.m. read newspaper	4	5
11–12 went for swim	5	9
12–1 p.m. lunch	3	5
1–3 p.m. shopping	5	8
4–5 p.m. tea with friend	4	9
5–6 p.m. prepare evening meal	3	4
6–7 p.m. eat with family	5	5
7–9 p.m. watch T.V with husband	3	8

Cognitive models of depression

Cognitive therapy is *defined* as a set of techniques used to alter maladaptive belief systems, attitudes and expectations. The two most widely accepted cognitive models for depression are:

1   Beck's model that depression is caused by negative thoughts about the self, about ongoing experience and the future (the so-called **cognitive triad**). See Fig. 12.2.
2   Seligman's model that depression is caused by the expectation of future helplessness, (the so-called 'helplessness model', Seligman, 1975). See Fig. 12.3.

In Beck's model there are said to be two mechanisms that produce depression the *cognitive triad* and *errors in logic*. The cognitive triad consists of three major cognitive patterns. The first of these is the patient's negative view of himself. He sees himself as inadequate, diseased and deprived. The second component is the depressed person's tendency to interpret ongoing experiences in a negative way. The third component is a tendency to take a negative view of the future: when the patient considers a task he expects to fail, and then anticipates that suffering and difficulty will continue forever.

The errors in logic in Beck's model fall into several categories. They are generally followed by *negative automatic thoughts* (**catastrophising negative automatic thoughts**). Learning how to identify negative automatic thoughts and deal with the errors in logic is at the heart of cognitive therapy for depression. Negative automatic thoughts are thoughts that 'pop into the head', that is they are difficult to control, and are *plausible* to the patient, hence difficult to challenge. They occur to a whole range of stimuli, so that patients develop a set of negative responses to everything and everybody around them, often including the therapist. Once a negative thought enters the head it cannot easily be dismissed, in this way having similarities to obsessive thoughts described in chapter 4.

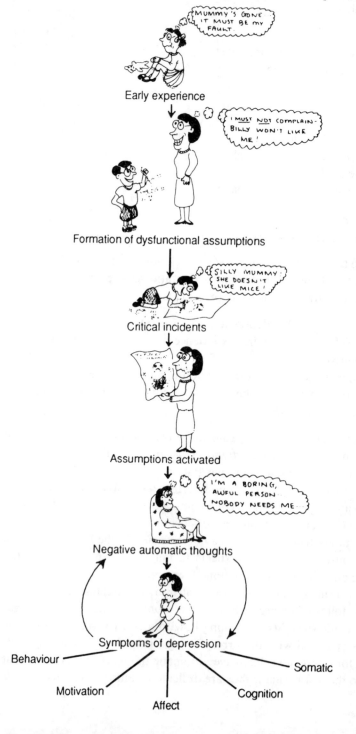

Fig. 12.2. Beck's cognitive model of depression.

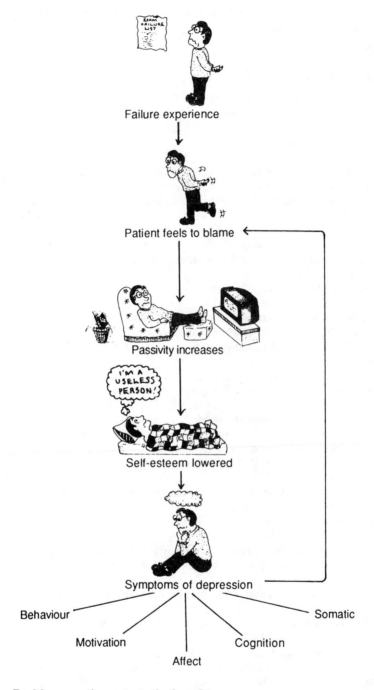

Failure experience

Patient feels to blame

Passivity increases

I'M A USELESS PERSON!

Self-esteem lowered

Symptoms of depression

Behaviour

Motivation

Affect

Cognition

Somatic

Fig. 12.3. Seligman's learned helplessness model.

Probing negative automatic thoughts

The aim here is for the therapist to teach the patient to re-evaluate their thinking. The emphasis has to be on what Beck has called '**collaborative empiricism**' and the use of the 'Socratic method'. In other words the therapist does not tell the patient that his thoughts are right or wrong, but develops a collaborative relationship with the patient to help challenge these beliefs and assess their validity.

The patient is asked:

1   What is the evidence for these thoughts?
2   Is there another way of looking at this?
3   Would it be better to look at this in a different way?

This is illustrated by a case example:

THERAPIST: Let us look at your diary of negative thoughts. Now what was actually going through your mind when you had these thoughts?

PATIENT: I start off thinking how my children have now grown up and really don't need me at all. Then it occurs to me what a boring person I am. Then as I sit there I feel how fat and ugly I am.

THERAPIST: Taking your first thought, can we see another way of explaining the facts, for instance can you think of some event in the last week where one of your children *did* need you?

PATIENT: My daughter asked me if her blouse matched her skirt yesterday . . . it's usually something trivial like that.

THERAPIST: Just a minute. There is another way of looking at this: let us suppose your daughter was really concerned about her appearance that day. She needed an opinion and valued yours. Can you think of anything to support what I have just said?

PATIENT: She was off to a party that night.

THERAPIST: So her appearance might have been very important to her, far from being trivial?

PATIENT: Well, I suppose you could be right.

THERAPIST: As a homework exercise could you think about it this way whenever your daughter asks you a question in future?

PATIENT: You mean say to myself- does she value my opinion?

THERAPIST: Yes, exactly!

THERAPIST: Now let us think about why you consider yourself to be so boring.

PATIENT: I certainly *was* boring, and I think I always will be.

THERAPIST: What is the evidence for this?

PATIENT: I have nothing to talk about.

THERAPIST: Let us consider this a minute. Is it really that you have nothing to say, or could it be that you do not consider yourself worth listening to?

PATIENT: Both!

THERAPIST: OK first of all, let us think about why you might not have much to talk about . . . Why could that be do you think?

PATIENT: Because I am stuck in the house all day, and I *do* nothing.

THERAPIST: So how could you change that?

PATIENT: Do something like evening classes, I suppose.

THERAPIST: Yes, that is an excellent idea. You would then have something different to talk about. Why do you think you are not worth listening to?

PATIENT: My husband falls asleep in the chair after his evening meal.

THERAPIST: Is there any other explanation possible for his behaviour?

PATIENT: He could be tired, I suppose.

THERAPIST: What evidence is there to support that.

PATIENT: He usually likes to take a nap after his meal. He did the same when we visited his mother.

THERAPIST: So it could be that if you tried conversing with him at a different time, it would be more effective. You can see how looking at things from a different point of view can be useful. Can you also use this approach with the feeling you have about your appearance?

(A similar technique was now used to examine the evidence that she was unattractive, find another way of looking at it, and see if she could agree that it was better to look at it this new way.)

Using this kind of dialogue, over a six session period of treatment, Mary gradually became able to generate alternative hypotheses for most of her unreasonable automatic thoughts. She was given a number of homework tasks, which included reading *Coping with Depression* by I. Blackburn and continuing to keep diaries of thoughts. One specific homework task was to write down a negative thought on one side of a sheet of paper, and a positive one gleaned from a treatment session on the other side: this has been described as the 'two-column technique'. Her Beck score for depression fell further, and she was clinically free of depression after eight sessions along these lines.

Probing errors of logic

Jane said 'I'm a complete failure in everything I do, I'm stuck here in this house with two young children, totally controlled by the situation, and can't do anything I want to. I'm bad tempered with the children, can't cook a decent meal or think of anything to say when my husband comes home from work'.

Jane went on to say how she had resented giving up work to look after her children, but felt her husband who was a successful solicitor, had all the things she wanted: power, prestige and the respect of others. To make matters worse she had just failed her driving test. She was 31 years old, and the children were 4 years and 18 months. When seen along with her husband it became clear just how much she resented his power and success, as this served to underline her own feelings of helplessness and inadequacy.

Jane was distorting her perception of reality in four *basic errors of logic* that are described by Beck:

1   **Arbitrary inference**. This happens when conclusions are drawn in an arbitrary way without really weighing up the evidence or considering alternatives. 'I'm a bad mother because I shout at the children' is an example of arbitrary inference.

2   **Selective abstraction**. There are many situations where we pay attention to some particular cues and ignore others, without doing so we would not be able to 'see the wood for the trees'. Depressed people pay attention selectively to the wrong cues, for instance, Jane concluded that her husband did not care about her because

when he came home from his busy solicitor's office he tended to tell her about his day, and often forgot to ask what she had been doing. She ignored the evidence of his caring for her, such as his regular buying of flowers, and kissing her on returning from work.

3   **Overgeneralisation**. If we are let down once by a friend we do not conclude immediately that the friend dislikes us, but usually think of other reasons why the friend let us down. Also when one person does let us down we do not jump to the conclusion that everybody else will do the same. When Jane felt let down about not passing her driving test, she said 'this just proves how hopeless and useless I am, I can never succeed in anything I do, I'm a born failure.'

4   **Magnification**. Here little things become totally out of proportion: often known colloquially as 'making a mountain out of a molehill'.

One day Jane burnt the evening meal. Her husband was not upset and volunteered to send out for some take away food, as they could not get a baby-sitter and go out for a meal. Jane reacted by blaming herself unduly, instead of accepting what happened as a mishap. She then refused to accept that their marriage had any future, and as there was nothing else to live for threatened to end her life.

In cognitive therapy Jane was encouraged to regard her beliefs and attitudes as though they were hypotheses that should be abandoned if they are found to be inadequate. She also needed to test out the alternative more adaptive beliefs that were generated.

The arbitrary inference about being a bad mother

THERAPIST: Do you think you are the only mother of two young children to shout at them?

JANE: I suppose not . . . but I don't hear other mothers shrieking all the time like I do.

THERAPIST: Fine, that may be so. Maybe you could test out how many other mothers of young children shout at them. How do you think you might do that?

JANE: Well, I suppose I could go to the mothers and toddlers group coffee mornings and see if they shout at their kids. I could also ask my best friend if she shouts at her children.

THERAPIST: Good, I would like you to put that into practice before our next session so we can discuss it then.

(At the next session Jane reported that she shouted about half as much as most other mothers. This evidence served to change her idea about being a bad mother.)

The selective abstraction that her husband did not care for her

THERAPIST: What is the evidence that your husband does not care for you?

JANE: He does not seem to be interested when I tell him things.

THERAPIST: OK, I can see you are disappointed in that, but let us suppose for the sake of argument that you are putting too much store by that. To support this argument can you tell me anything else he does which might mean he cares?

JANE: He usually brings me flowers, and I get a kiss on the cheek when he comes in from work.

THERAPIST: Now that sounds to me as if you are not really paying attention to his behaviour overall.

Jane was then given the homework task of trying to think as much as possible about the evidence for her husband loving her during the next week, and to write down such activity when it occurs and bring the list to the next session. She did report that this served to reduce the time spent thinking about his lack of conversational attention.

Overgeneralisation that she was a born failure

Recently, the final straw for Jane was when she failed her driving test, as this served to confirm her hypothesis that she was a failure.

THERAPIST: Do you think everyone passes their driving test first time?

JANE: No, I suppose not, but my husband did.

THERAPIST: So if you cannot compete with him this means you are a failure?

JANE: I see what you mean. If I compare myself with him I am bound to look pathetic especially in areas where he excels – he has an advanced drivers certificate. The woman next door has failed her test four times, but I just assume I will fail again on the next attempt so I might as well give up now.

THERAPIST: Have you heard of any other people failing their test first time?

JANE: Yes, now I come to think of it there is Mrs B. and also Mrs. C.

THERAPIST: So in fact lots of people fail the test first time. What is the evidence that you will fail next time?

JANE: Well there isn't any. My instructor is hopeful, and was surprised when I failed last time.

Magnification of a burnt meal into a disaster

THERAPIST: What did you say to *yourself* when you burnt the meal?

JANE: That is it . . . I can't cope with another thing . . . my husband will really think me pathetic . . . give up . . . I even thought of killing myself though I know that's ridiculous.

THERAPIST: What did your husband actually say?

JANE: Let us see if we can get a baby-sitter and go out to eat. But we could not get one, so that was it as far as I was concerned. He tried to persuade me that he could bring in some take-away food, but I just felt it was too hopeless.

THERAPIST: What do you feel about it now?

JANE: I can see that I made a mountain out of a molehill. I should not have let things get out of hand.

THERAPIST: The important thing is to learn from this experience, and the next time small things get out of proportion, could you try and remember this session?

Other cognitive techniques

Probing dysfunctional assumptions

Beck has derived from Horney (1950) the notion that some patients become depressed because of *rules* or *assumptions* that they consider to be absolutely true in all situations, and these rules become part of their cognitive structure. Such patients judge themselves inadequate compared to their own high standards.

After her husband left her, Betty decided to devote her energies to her three school-age children, who lived with her. She decided that she had to deliver each child to school each day and collect them herself. She was aged 41 years and a former secretary, but had not worked since her marriage at the age of 22 years. She had strong feelings about the fact that her ex-husband had remarried a woman half his age, and also felt angry because her ex-husband would take the children for the weekend whenever it suited him. When asked what she thought about this she said 'I do not think I *should* complain or my ex-husband will not like it, and the children might suffer'. She had been divorced for five years and had the chance of making a new relationship, but said 'I would like to, but I don't think I *should*, the children might not like it'.

Treatment
Role reversal

Betty was asked to imagine she was her ex-husband, and to imagine what goes through his mind when he asks for the children at the weekend, and she said 'he would think that I am so insipid and uninteresting that the children must find me very dull, they would *rather* be with him'

THERAPIST: Have you ever *asked* the children whether this is true, and what they would prefer to do at the weekend?
PATIENT: No, I thought I *shouldn't* do that, but perhaps you have got a point.

Examination of when 'shoulds' apply and to what degree

Betty was asked to examine the situations in her life where 'shoulds' apply and gradually a list was developed where the rule 'you should't say how you are dissatisfied or the children won't like you' applied. This included such things as telling the children when to switch off the TV, and having a relationship with her boyfriend. The different degrees to which her rule applied in these situations gradually became apparent to her.

Catching the patient talking in 'shoulds' in treatment

Examples have been given of how Betty's talk was dominated by 'shoulds'. She used the word frequently, and each time she did so this was pointed out to her. She was given the homework task of keeping a list of the number of times she told herself what to do in this kind of way.

Comparison of the 'shoulds' with what the patient really wants

Betty's life was so dominated by 'shoulds' she rarely satisfied her own needs. At the end of six sessions devoted to the above three techniques, she was able to realise that it was allowable to have needs of her own. It then became clearer to her that she needed to stand up to her ex-husband over the question of access to her children at weekends. After two more sessions, she was also able to see that she could have a boyfriend, because this is what she really wanted.

Cognitive-expectancy techniques

Depressed patients often blame themselves when things go wrong even when events are beyond their control. This can be explained using the second cognitive model of depression the **learned helpless** model (Seligman, 1975). It is cognitive because it states that the basic cause of depression is an expectation: the patient expects that bad events will occur and there is nothing he or she can do to prevent their occurrence. Evidence suggests that when patients fail at important tasks and make internal explanations for their failure, passivity appears and self-esteem drops. When individuals make external explanations for failure, passivity ensues but self-esteem stays high (Abramson, Seligman & Teasdale, 1978).

Seligman argues that a useful way of intervening in depression is at the end rather than at the beginning of a presumed causal chain, and specifically interventions should be directed at *expectations*. This is known as the **cognitive-expectancy technique**. An example of this model in action is given below:

Sarah was a 34-year-old bank clerk who had become profoundly depressed after an incident in the bank when a customer had asked for some information about his account which Sarah could not find. It had been a hectic day at the bank and when she wrote down the customer's account number she had accidentally reversed two of the digits, and so the computer could not find the account. The customer shouted at her, Sarah blushed and because she felt so ashamed could not face any more customers that day. She stayed at home for two weeks persuading her doctor that she had influenza. She later admitted this was not the case but she could not face going to work in case she made a similar mistake. When she did return to work she went 'off sick' again and it was at this stage she was seen for cognitive therapy.

Formulation of onset of depression

Sarah could have made any number of explanations for not returning to work. The first time she invoked a medical explanation 'I am sick', but the second time she said to herself 'I am incompetent'. Furthermore she believed her incompetence was not just related to the one episode:

'Because I am incompetent, I will make another silly mistake at work'. Sarah was convinced that her one failure proved that she was generally incompetent, and would fail if she returned to her job *also* she would fail at any other job she applied for. This made her profoundly depressed.

When Sarah thought of going back to work the second time, her belief in her incompetence led to the formulation of a negative expectation, namely that even if she tried again at work she would fail again. She now firmly expected not to succeed and so refused to go back to work. Her non-activity now guaranteed her non-success.

Treatment
PATIENT: I made a mistake with those numbers, people in my job are not supposed
        to do that. I am expected *never* to make a mistake. I know I will make a
        mistake again so why try?
THERAPIST: You did fail *once* it is clear, but how can you be so sure you will fail
        again?
PATIENT: It will happen again and there is nothing I can do about it . . . I suppose
        that is what I keep saying to myself.
THERAPIST: And how does that make you feel?
PATIENT: Hopeless. Also depressed.
THERAPIST: You cannot know for sure that you will be unable to cope unless you
        try, maybe it is not totally hopeless.

This kind of dialogue, carried out over six sessions in which Sarah was encouraged to look at events in a different way is similar in many respects to Beck's cognitive therapy. 'Collaborative empiricism' and the 'Socratic approach' are used in both cases although the therapist here is helping the patient feel better despite the perceived deficits, rather than exploring the validity of the perception.

By gaining objectivity in this way Sarah could become less self reproaching, and she had identified the cause of the problem as being outside of herself. This technique is particularly valuable in patients like Sarah who was prone to excessive self-blame, and always assumed the responsibility when anything went wrong.

An important next step was to encourage Sarah back to work, she was reluctant to do this and had to accept that even if it did not wor)at she had nothing to lose by trying. She came to see her therapist afte₁ the first week back at work and said: 'Perhaps I coped with the first week because I am not so bad at it after all, perhaps I am not so incompetent.'

The cognitive-expectancy theory of change had a clear role in the case described, although as indicated it is often part of the general management of depression, being used along with other cognitive and behavioural techniques.

Specific techniques for suicidal wishes

In many parts of the UK the most common reason why women are admitted to a general hospital is because of self-injurious behaviour, and it is also the second most common reason for men to be admitted. For some of these cases a cognitive- behavioural approach is *not* indicated, for example those cases where biological depression or physical illness are implicated. However in many cases the self-injurious behaviour can be seen as an impulsive act carried out to produce some kind of response from their circle of contacts. The purpose of the behaviour is to alter their life situation not to die, and it is in this kind of case where a behavioural approach can prove valuable:

Case illustration

Roberta was 22 years old, and she lived at home with parents with whom she had an uneasy truce. Her parents disapproved of her life-style in every way and she seemed to do everything possible to contradict their 'middle-class' values. She spent her time with a peer group that rode around the neighbourhood on motor scooters, and her boyfriend was a member of this gang. After her boyfriend had been prosecuted for minor drug offences her parents forbade her to see him again, and she took her first overdose which consisted of a handful of her mother's sleeping tablets. The family discord was not resolved however, and so she took another more serious overdose some weeks later resulting in a period of assessment in a psychiatric unit. Her parents gathered round her bedside in great concern, and family therapy sessions were instituted. On week-end leave Roberta took another overdose of tablets. When this was discussed with her she said: 'I'll take an overdose each time I'm dis-charged.'

Formulation
Roberta had learnt to cope with a difficult situation by indulging in potentially dangerous behaviour. Each time she did this she had been rewarded by concern from her family and a great deal of attention from the medical profession. Family therapy was not having any immediate effect and there was an increasing danger to her life.

Treatment
At this point it was decided to try to change the reinforcement contingen-cies: we wanted to reinforce Roberta for *therapeutic* not anti-therapeutic behaviour. She was therefore told that in future she would never be admitted to the psychiatric unit if she had taken an overdose or injured herself in anyway. She would of course receive the necessary *medical* treatment but would then be discharged home. On the other hand she was told that if she asked for our help she would be seen promptly by a member of the team. After she had been seen in this way, family therapy sessions were also made contingent on *not* taking an overdose. In this way the family were gradually made aware that they needed to show

concern for Roberta *other* than at times when she had taken an overdose. When this concern was exploited in family sessions it was possible to deal with parental disapproval of her boyfriend, and the self-injurious behaviour ceased.

Cognitive techniques for suicidal wishes

Suicidal patients often feel hopeless, seeing themselves trapped in an insoluble problem. They will often say: 'I cannot change the situation; so there is no point in living.' This was the case with John, a 70-year-old man whose wife had discovered that he had written some flirtatious letters to another woman some years ago and had now threatened to leave him. They were in fact very happily married, and he had never been unfaithful to his wife. However, when she threatened to leave him, he could see no way out except to end his life and he took a very serious overdose of tablets. When interviewed after he had recovered with extensive medical treatment, a cognitive technique was used to try to show the *logical inconsistencies* in his belief systems:

THERAPIST: Why did you take the overdose of tablets?
JOHN: I could not imagine life without Barbara. (His wife's name)
THERAPIST: Why did you feel there was no hope of you and Barbara getting together again?
JOHN: It was such a wicked thing I did . . . those letters . . . I do not expect she will ever forgive . . .
THERAPIST: What is the evidence that she will never forgive you?
JOHN: I do not have any, but I know I can't live without Barbara.
THERAPIST: Just a minute. Is there anything that has happened to contradict that?
JOHN: She did visit me yesterday.
THERAPIST: How did the meeting go?
JOHN: She was very forgiving; so it is possible you could be right. There might be a chance.
THERAPIST: What do you rate your chances are of getting back together now?

At this stage it was felt that a 'cognitive breakthrough' had been made, and John was soon discharged from hospital. They were seen together for follow-up and it was clear that the improvement had been maintained. As in this case, it is important to discuss the reason for suicidal wishes, and why the patient sees suicide as the only escape from a miserable or intolerable life situation. Often a patient has suicidal thoughts that a life situation cannot be changed, when in fact it can. Careful probing and a re-examination of the situation can produce a cognitive shift, although it is often more time-consuming and more difficult than the case described.

Specific techniques where depression is part of a grief reaction

Grief is the typical response to bereavement, and in most cases is the normal response. Freud (1917) has described the value of mourning in helping the bereaved come to terms with loss. However, in some cases grief becomes abnormal, and in these cases the preoccupation with mourning continues for a prolonged period, there may even be perceptual disturbances, for example auditory and visual pseudo-hallucinations, and behavioural changes, for example clinging to objects that belonged to the deceased, and features usually associated with depression, for example lack of interest, guilty feelings, loss of energy, along with sleep and appetite disturbances. Other psychiatric disorders may also be mimicked.

Behavioural and cognitive treatments for abnormal grief derive from a variety of sources, for example Ramsay (1977), and Gauthier & Marshall (1977). A series of cases have been studied by Liebermann (1978), Mawson *et al.* (1981) and Sireling, Cohen & Marks (1988). The approach of **guided mourning** likens unresolved grief to other forms of phobic avoidance, where the treatment is *exposure* to the avoided situation as described in chapter 3. In guided mourning patients are encouraged to expose themselves repeatedly to avoided cognitive, affective and behavioural cues concerning bereavement, for example facing the distressing situation of the crematorium which had been previously avoided as in the following case:

Case illustration

Mrs H., who was 65 years old, had suffered from a variety of symptoms for seven years, since the death of her mother, to whom she was very close. Most prominent was a feeling of tension and anxiety, and an inability to control the shaking of her right arm. She also had 'a black feeling of depression like a cloud hanging over me', along with difficulty getting off to sleep and a poor appetite. She had lost interest in all her former hobbies, and recently had lost interest in almost everything so that she tended to remain alone in a darkened room.

On closer questioning about her mother, it transpired that she had nursed her through her terminal illness. In this illness her mother had a stroke in which her *right arm* had gone into convulsive movements. When the link was made between her mother's symptom and her own Mrs H. admitted 'you could be right I'd never thought of that'. Mrs H. attended the funeral but made the revealing remark 'I was too upset at the time to feel much, I had to concentrate on making all the arrangements, and I couldn't cry in front of all those people'. The details were that her mother had been cremated because that was her mother's wish, and when the undertaker had asked Mrs H. what she wished done with the ashes she had told him to dispose of them, as she herself was too disturbed to make up her mind what to do.

Pre-treatment assessment showed an elevated Beck depression score of 24 (moderate depression) and the *formulation* was that this patient's depression was due to the fact that she had avoided facing the sad feelings at the time of her mother's death, hence had remained depressed. The symptom in this patient's arm is reminiscent of the famous case of Anna O. from the pschoanalytic literature (Freud, 1955), where Freud described mourning as the reaction to the loss of a loved person. However, in place of a psychodynamic explanation, we can equally explain the symptom in *cognitive* and *behavioural* terms: Mrs H. had her attention focused on her right arm when nursing her dying mother and so discomfort and her right arm become associated. Whenever she felt tension subsequently it was her right arm that manifested symptoms. She had not been able to express her grief at the time of the funeral and this cognitive avoidance had been continued. Subsequently the crematorium meant little to her because there was no place she could think of as associated with her mother, that is it had developed into behavioural avoidance.

Treatment

A therapeutic *contract* was made with Mrs H. in which she agreed to attend for six sessions at an agreed frequency which was once every two weeks. This interval was chosen so that she would have time to carry out agreed homework tasks.

In the first session the therapist explained the features of healthy grief and why the patient's grief was unhealthy, and reviewed the events prior to her mother's death. She was helped to understand how *not* facing up to sad feelings at the time of her mother's death was related to her symptoms. As with phobic patients, it is often useful to explain how avoidance leads to difficulties later on: 'If you fall off a bicycle, then the best thing is to get back on right away. The longer you wait the more difficult it will be for you to ride again. You did not face the sad feelings about your mother at the time, because it was so painful, and that was understandable, but now you can see the importance of facing these feelings as soon as possible'.

In the second session she discussed ways that she might be able to face the loss at this late stage, the problem being that the crematorium meant little to her. As a homework exercise, she was asked to try to think of a way to overcome this problem, and decided to arrange a memorial to her mother. This was to be a rose planted in the garden of remembrance or a seat in the garden of remembrance, with a plaque bearing an inscription to her mother.

At the third session, she reported that she had decided on the rose and had gone ahead with these arrangements. Some discussion followed about what she ought to write on the memorial plaque near the rose. At the fourth session she was tearful when describing how upset she had been on visiting the garden of remembrance, and she was praised for expressing feelings in this way. She was made to feel that it was perfectly acceptable to cry when thinking about her mother. On the remaining sessions it was stressed that she should visit the garden of remembrance at least once a week, and remain for at least an hour to help her express the sad feelings.

At the end of treatment the Beck depression score was 5, and she was free of all major symptoms. Follow up at two years showed the improvement to be maintained, and she was visiting the garden of remembrance at appropriate times only: the anniversary of her mother's death and the anniversary of her mother's birthday.

Several other techniques can be used in conjunction with guided mourning, and these include:

> Saying goodbye: here the patient is encouraged to role-play a situation in which they imagine the deceased person to be sitting in the room with them and they 'say goodbye' and take the opportunity to express things they may not have been able to before. Bringing photographs of the deceased may assist here.
>
> Writing a letter to the deceased person, and bringing the letter to a therapy session and reading it aloud to the photograph.
>
> Spending agreed periods of time in a bedroom formerly occupied by the deceased, and/or wearing objects of clothing or jewellery that belonged to the deceased.
>
> Making a list of the positive and negative attributes of the deceased. The aim here is to bring out any avoided emotions such as anger, guilt and painful memories.

Summary

- Depression is a complex condition having biological, behavioural and cognitive components. It is, therefore, not surprising that multi-modal treatments involving behavioural and cognitive approaches have been found to be effective.
- Behavioural techniques focus on increasing activity level, reducing unwanted behaviour, inducing emotions not compatible with depression, and increasing the patients skills.
- Specific behavioural approaches include teaching 'mastery' and 'pleasure'.
- Cognitive models of depression by Beck and Seligman are described.
- Beck's model leads to treatment of negative automatic thoughts, and the correction of logical errors such as: arbitrary influence, selective abstraction, overgeneralisation and magnification.
- Seligman's learned helplessness model leads to treatment by the use of cognitive-expectancy changing techniques.
- There are some specific approaches both behavioural and cognitive for patients with suicidal ideas.
- Abnormal grief can be treated by guided mourning which is a variant of exposure therapy.

13 Behavioural medicine

Behavioural medicine is the application of behavioural and cognitive therapy to medicine. One group of applications consists of those conditions where psychiatry has had a traditional application in medicine, formerly known as *psychosomatic medicine*. These include: asthma, eczema and duodenal ulcer. In these conditions there is usually some organic pathology, but there is thought to be a psychological cause. The second group of conditions are those formerly known as *hypochondriasis*, and more recently as **illness behaviour**. This is where psychological factors are thought to be the reason for the maintenance of the behaviour which then manifests as illness. There is also probably a *third* group where the picture is complicated and it is debatable whether organic pathology exists or not.

Whether the condition falls into one of these three groups is nowadays not important from the point of view of psychological therapy. It was important, however, when the field of psychosomatic medicine was dominated by psychoanalysis. The principal of treatment today is to assess the patient's symptoms from a psychological point of view, after reasonable attempts have been made to exclude medical pathology, bearing in mind that a condition that might have started out with an organic cause is now maintained by psychological factors.

Recently, an exciting new theory has developed a model of hypochondriasis or illness behaviour as being similar to obsessive-compulsive disorder. In their work, Salkovskis & Warwick (1986) suggest that the thought of illness is comparable to an obsessional idea which intrudes on consciousness and leads to increased anxiety. Instead of the patient trying to reduce this anxiety by rituals, in hypochondriasis the patient seeks medical reassurance. Each time such reassurance is given, the anxiety reduces a small amount but then doubt creeps in and further reassurance is required. Thus medical reassurance helps to maintain the anxiety in the same way that rituals and reassurance maintain anxiety in obsessive-compulsive disorder (see Fig. 13.1).

Using their model, Salkovskis & Warwick suggest that treatment should consist of the following components:

1   Education of patient.
2   A ban on medical reassurance.

3   Cognitive restructuring to alter faulty beliefs.
4   Behavioural testing of hypotheses.

These components of treatment are demonstrated by Salkovskis & Warwick (1986) in two case histories but a controlled trial of this treatment is being performed at the time of writing this chapter. The use of a similar technique applied to groups of patients has also been described (Barsky, A. J., 1989).

The following case illustrates these techniques.

Case illustration of illness behaviour

Susan, a 31-year-old librarian was referred to the clinic by her GP with a three-year history of excessive anxiety about her health with a preoccupation that she might have breast cancer.

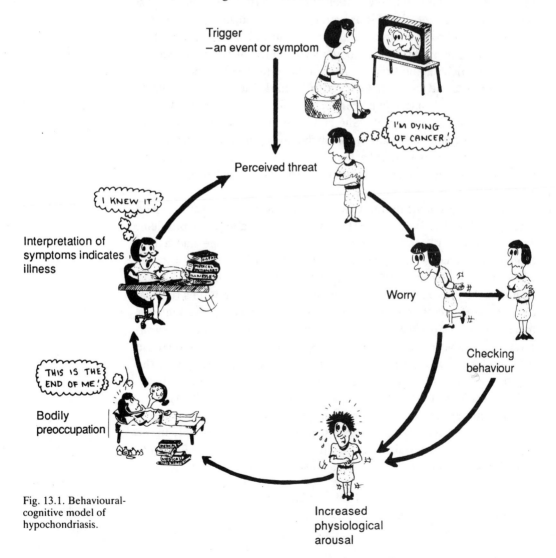

Fig. 13.1. Behavioural-cognitive model of hypochondriasis.

Her anxiety had started after she had watched a television programme which discussed the role of mammography in 'well woman' screening clinics. Following this, Susan had examined her breasts and thought she felt a small lump. She returned to her doctor again who this time found a small nodule which he felt was benign but agreed to Susan being referred for mammography. The mammography had been normal but, at Susan's insistence, she had been referred for a surgical opinion. The surgeon reluctantly agreed to perform a biopsy. The biopsy results suggested a benign fibrous adenoma and no further investigations were indicated. Susan, however failed to be convinced of the lack of serious pathology. Since that time she visited her GP's surgery at least once a week with a series of complaints which she believed were evidence of breast cancer. These had included tracheitis which she believed was evidence of cancerous invasion of her chest, and headaches which she felt were due to secondary brain tumours. She had changed her GP twice over the past three years due to her lack of satisfaction with their diagnoses. Every day she performed breast examinations six to eight times to ensure that no further lumps had appeared, and she spent much of her time reading books and articles about breast cancer in the library where she worked.

Her personal and family history were unremarkable. A maternal uncle had died of bowel cancer five years earlier but otherwise there was no history of cancer in the family. She had been married to John for eight years and there were no children although they intended to start a family in two or three years time. Her marriage was happy apart from John's irritation with her constant inquiries of whether he believed she had cancer.

In the first session the therapist obtained a history from Susan and then suggested that they both had different hypotheses about the problem. The therapist explained that whereas Susan believed she had a life-threatening cancer, the therapist believed she had an anxiety disorder which was causing a number of distressing symptoms and which was maintained by her seeking medical reassurance, seeking John's reassurance, reading excessively about cancer and by constantly checking her breasts. It was hardly surprising that Susan could not accept the therapist's view of the situation, but she did agree to test this theory over the next week by recording her anxiety at hourly intervals throughout the day, and before and after she engaged in a reassurance seeking activity.

Susan returned to the second session with her diary of anxiety completed. Although she still could not accept that she did not have cancer, she had noticed that her reassurance seeking reduced her anxiety in the short-term but that it quickly recurred. In view of this, she reluctantly agreed that over the next month she would:

1   Not attend her GP or medical practitioner other than her behavioural psychotherapist.

2   Not request reassurance from John. John was instructed to answer all such requests by saying, 'I'm afraid I've been asked by the clinic not to answer questions like that'.

3   Not to read any articles or books about cancer. To make this easier for her, Susan agreed to use any free time in the library in researching the origins of Stone Age monuments in Britain, a subject which particularly interested her, and to give the therapist an essay on this at the next meeting.

4   Not to perform breast examination. To make this easier, Susan agreed not to wait until the other librarians had left at lunch and coffee times so that she could go into the washrooms unobserved but to go for lunch and coffee with her colleagues. In the evenings, instead of examining her breasts following a bath, John would stay with her and encourage her not to perform breast examination. Usually she would also go upstairs and examine her breasts several times during an evening, and John was asked to encourage and praise her for *not* doing this.

Susan managed to comply with most of these instructions and at the third session, a week later reported that her level of tension was already less although she was still convinced that she was dying of cancer.

The therapist then started to explain the principles of *cognitive therapy*. The basic methods of cognitive therapy have already been explained in relation to anxiety and depression in chapters 11 and 12 of this book. In this case, Susan's underlying maladaptive assumption was that she had cancer of the breast, which was unrecognised by the medical practitioners she had consulted, and it was spreading to cause a variety of symptoms which would ultimately lead to her demise. The next step was for Susan to recognise the *negative automatic thoughts* which linked with this assumption, and which resulted in her symptoms of anxiety.

The idea of negative automatic thoughts was explained:

When anyone starts to feel anxious there are thoughts which pass through your mind which lead to that anxiety. These thoughts often occur very quickly and may lead to a sequence of thoughts that seem to verify your belief that you are dying of cancer. For example, you might be sitting at work after lunch and you experience a sudden mild pain in your abdomen. Your first thought might be 'I've got a pain in my stomach – it must be due to the cancer', this thought might be closely followed by visions of yourself visiting a cancer specialist who tells you that you are dying, and finally by a mental picture of yourself on your death bed with John crying over you. Because you have had the pain, you automatically ignore any other explanations of the pain but assume that it is evidence for your belief that you are dying of cancer. Understandably, these thoughts make you feel very anxious and miserable. The anxiety itself will tend to cause you to experience more bodily symptoms, which again you construe as symptoms of cancer.

Please monitor and record these negative automatic thoughts, which come into your mind and lead to the anxiety-provoking thought sequence. Write these thoughts down together with a rating on a scale of 0–100 as to how much you believe them to be true. Then I want you to write down all the evidence for and any evidence against the thought. For example, in the situation described before the negative automatic thought was:

'I have a pain in my stomach – it must be cancer'.

The evidence for this might be:

'People with cancer may sometimes have pains in their stomach.'

The evidence against might be:

'I have just eaten a large lunch and the pain is mild, it is most likely to be due to my eating too much too quickly.'

'People with cancer often do not complain of pain.'

'I have been extensively investigated and none of the doctors can find any evidence that I have cancer, so it is unlikely that I have advanced secondaries causing abdominal pain.'

Susan was then told:

After you have weighed up all the evidence, I would like you to put another rating from 0–100 of your belief in the negative automatic thought.

Susan complied with these instructions, and apart from some initial difficulty in examining the evidence for her belief dispassionately, progressed well. The next six sessions were spent with the therapist looking at Susan's weekly thought diaries and then choosing any particular areas of difficulty and examining them with her during the session. For example, at the fifth session, Susan reported that she had irrefutable evidence that she might be dying of cancer. She had discovered a lump in her groin, and was sure that this was cancer and could not think of any alternative explanations. The therapist asked her if she had ever heard of anyone having any lumps in the groin at all that were not cancer. After a long pause, Susan reported that she herself had once had a lump in the groin as a child which had proved to be due to an infected hair follicle. She then volunteered that the lump she had now was red, painful and hot to touch and was thus similar in nature to the previous lump. After saying this, Susan said that she had read that the enlargement of lymph nodes found in cancer patients was normally painless. Her belief in this finding being absolute proof of her dying of cancer reduced from 100 per cent certain to less that 10 per cent during the session. Following this session, Susan was set the task of testing out her beliefs about the lump. She was asked to visit her GP, and to ask him to examine the lump, but not to seek any reassurance other than this, and not to use any words associated with cancer during the visit.

At the end of eight sessions, Susan's belief that she was dying of cancer was reduced to less than five per cent. She no longer had the urge to examine her breasts, did not seek reassurance from her husband or GP and had no urge to actively seek out books on cancer. In view of this improvement, she was asked to continue with her thought diaries only when she had any thoughts which she could not rationalise without writing them down. Arrangements were made for her to be followed up in the clinic but active treatment was stopped. By six-month post treatment follow-up she had managed to reintroduce *monthly* self examination of her breasts without any increase of her anxiety symptoms.

This case illustrates many of the principals involved in behavioural medicine, and these principals can be applied to a wide range of disorders, some of these disorders being common well known syndromes, for example irritable bowel syndrome, others being symptoms with an associated pathology, for example diabetes related to overeating. The list of conditions to which behavioural medicine can be applied is as large as medicine itself. In order to illustrate the main principals the following conditions are described in the rest of this chapter:

> Irritable bowel
> Irritable bladder
> Compulsive cough
> Resistant asthma
> Hypertension
> Diabetes related to overeating
> Epilepsy
> Abdominal pain
> Vomiting fear
> Insomnia

Irritable bowel syndrome

Irritable bowel syndrome (IBS) is defined as abdominal pain and a change in bowel habit, which may be diarrhoea *or* constipation, in the absence of any organic pathology. A behavioural model has been proposed which assumes that IBS involves symptomatic changes in bowel habits which are unlearned responses to stressful circumstances (Latimer, 1981). This model goes on to suggest that idiosyncratic learning of maladaptive coping then takes place due to:

1   Misconceptions about 'normal' bowel habits.
2   Learning that symptoms of IBS are socially acceptable.
3   Learning that symptoms of IBS are a way of avoiding something unpleasant.
4   Learning that symptoms of IBS are a way of eliciting concern from others.

If the symptomatic change in bowel habits is *unlearned* it makes sense to direct therapy at the maladaptive coping which has been learnt. It follows from this that the goal is *not* complete elimination of symptoms, since the elimination of all stress is not practicable.

Case illustration

'I have had diarrhoea for 17 years, and it totally dominates my life', said a pleasant 45-year-old lady referred to us by a general physician. The physician had carried out extensive investigations, but nothing abnormal had been discovered. She said the diarrhoea began after a holiday abroad, and she probably had had a genuine bowel infection at that time. However, over the years she has increased the amount of medication she takes to attempt to lower bowel motility, so that she was now taking vast amounts, claiming that she could not leave the house unless she did so 'in case of an accident'. One year ago she gave up work altogether, because she claimed this entailed going too far from a toilet.

In her past it was noted that she had had mild attacks of diarrhoea before taking examinations. She had never married, but had a reasonably active social life, and claimed that she used to enjoy her work as a secretary, before the symptoms forced her to give it up.

She suffered from abdominal discomfort, as well as an anxiety that she would lose control of her bowels. The anxiety lead to more abdominal discomfort, and hence ever increasing fears of what might happen 'in case of an accident'.

Treatment

This patient had already tried to help herself by attending to dietary factors. She had also tried psychotherapy and hypnotherapy to no avail. In the early sessions of behavioural-cognitive therapy she was introduced to the concept of learning coping strategies:

THERAPIST: What is the main way that your problem of irritable bowel interferes with your life?

PATIENT: It means I can't go anywhere unless I have easy access to a private lavatory.

THERAPIST: What would happen if you were caught out, and had to use a public lavatory?

PATIENT: I would be anxious that people would notice me, and I would be embarrassed. The thing is I know it would take me a long time in the lavatory, and if I could hear other people outside wanting to use it then I would get more anxious.

THERAPIST: What would be so terrible if you kept others waiting?

PATIENT: I'm not sure.

THERAPIST: Could it be that you have exaggerated the importance of what others might think? Perhaps we could work out a way of putting this to the test.

With this kind of discussion the patient was persuaded to try a **behavioural experiment** and venture out to use a public lavatory. In the event she found it was possible to do so, despite the continued need to visit the lavatory too often. Next she was taught *relaxation exercises* which were tape recorded for her so that she could practice this at home, and another homework exercise was for her to keep a record, in diary form, of the frequency of visits to the lavatory. The diaries were discussed in subsequent sessions, and she was asked to carry out the further behavioural experiment of waiting for 10 minutes before actually emptying her bowels. She found this task possible at first only if she was sitting on the lavatory seat, but later on was gradually able to postpone the visits to the lavatory.

At the end of 12 sessions over a 30-week period, the distress associated with her problem was greatly reduced. She was able to resume her secretarial job, which in turn boosted her confidence. She remained with a considerable problem of diarrhoea, but the gradual improvement and the changes in her life-style were thought by the patient to be well worth while.

It is often the case in behavioural medicine that a cure is not possible. Nevertheless, by adopting the kind of approach used in this case relatively small improvements in symptoms can bring about great changes in the quality of life. For this reason the techniques described are often valuable in individual cases, despite the fact that one controlled study of behavioural therapy for irritable bowel syndrome showed little advantage for behavioural interventions over standard medical management (Newell, R., 1989).

Irritable bladder (detrusor instability)

Detrusor instability is a condition in which the detrusor (bladder) muscle is shown objectively to contract spontaneously when the bladder is filling. In itself this condition may be asymptomatic, or may lead to *frequency* or *nocturia*. Frequency is usually defined as the passage of urine in excess of every two hours, or 7 times, during the waking day. Nocturia is the arousal from sleep twice or more every night to void. Macaulay *et al.* (1987) carried out a controlled trial of psychotherapy, behavioural treatment and medication in 50 patients with detrusor instability. The intriguing results suggested that psychotherapy was best for nocturia, but behavioural treatment was best for frequency. The following case illustrates the behavioural approach.

Case illustration

Sarah was referred by her gynaecologist who did not think she would benefit from surgery for her symptom of frequency of micturition, despite having the condition known as 'detrusor instability'. She was greatly inconvenienced by the problem because her job as a high pressured salesperson involved attending meetings, and prolonged car travel, both of which were often interrupted to visit the lavatory.

'I realise it's worse when I'm under stress, but I'm not sure exactly what it is that brings it on' she said. She had a vague idea that alcohol and coffee made it worse. Most of her life seemed well organised, however, and she had coped with a divorce, and organised her two children to be looked after by a full-time nanny. She very much enjoyed her job, and was successful despite having a male dominated career.

One of the principles of behavioural medicine is to ask the patient to *self-monitor* as much as possible.   At the end of the first session she was asked to keep a 'urinary diary', which is a simple record of how many times she needed to pass water each day, along with comments about stress factors during the day, and a record of how much coffee and alcohol she had consumed.

Treatment

Sarah brought her urinary diary to the next session, and several facts emerged: whenever she was tired and fatigued through lack of sleep the symptoms were worse, and they were also exacerbated by alcohol and coffee. She agreed to cut out alcohol altogether, and went over to decaffeinated coffee. She also agreed to go to bed no later than 12 midnight. These changes brought about an immediate improvement in symptoms, the frequency of micturition was reduced from 15–18 times per day to 8–11 times per day. This was itself reinforcing, because she could see immediate results which more than made up for the deprivation of coffee and alcohol. She was also very keen to continue the urinary diary.

Further sessions were spent analyzing the urinary diaries, and it became clear that when she felt tense she was more likely to pass water. Passing water gave her a feeling of relief, and so was itself reinforcing.

Relaxation training

In discussion with Sarah it became clear to her that at the times when she was tense she was likely to feel the need to pass water. She was then taught some simple relaxation exercises to practice at home. When she had become skilled in these she was to use the relaxation as a means of anxiety reduction *instead* of going to the lavatory to pass water.

In teaching relaxation skills the first point is for the patient to understand the need to acquire these skills and to see how it relates to symptom-relief. The self monitoring had been the key to this in Sarah's case. Next it has to be assumed, that in our culture at least, relaxation is not something that comes naturally to most people, so it follows that relaxation has to be *learnt*. The technique of relaxation training is described in the Appendix 1.

An important homework exercise was for her to practice the relaxation at home each day by playing the tape that had been made for her. Later on she was asked to carry out the *behavioural test* similar to the previous case: she was asked to postpone passing water by at least 10 minutes, using her relaxation exercise to help her do this. At the end of 10 session of therapy along these lines this patient was able to reduce the frequency of micturition to five or six times in an average day. This satisfactory outcome meant that her life was no longer seriously impaired by the bladder symptoms.

Compulsive cough

Case illustration

A middle-aged man was referred because the physician treating him could not relieve the patient's anxieties about coughing up sputum. The patient had been treated for many years for chest infections which did indeed cause him to bring up sputum, but this was now confined to the winter months, and always responded to short courses of antibiotics. However, the patient was constantly preoccupied with the feeling that he had some sputum at the back of his throat, and had taken to carrying around a small plastic sputum pot to spit out the sputum should the need arise.

Behavioural formulation

The sputum pot served to reduce his anxiety, and he would not go anywhere without it. He had previously been reinforced with praise for using the sputum pot by his physician, and he had associated the use of the sputum pot with this praise. This had been reinforced in the past when it's use had been both necessary and important, for instance when sputum was needed to test for antibiotic sensitivity. He now had acquired a conditioned response: the stimulus was the feeling of sputum at the back of the throat, and this caused the response of bringing out the sputum pot which he always kept handy.

Treatment

After some discussion with the physician in charge of the case it was agreed to tell the patient that the sputum pot was no longer necessary, and the patient was urged to throw it away, which he did with great difficulty. He was then taught relaxation exercises, in the same way as in the previous case (Sarah) to use each time he felt the need to cough up sputum, but he still remained anxious and distressed. Finally an *exposure* technique was used: he was taught to tolerate having a small amount of sputum in his mouth, and then to swallow it rather than cough it up. This produced high anxiety in the initial sessions, but after six sessions the anxiety was minimal. He was reassured that during the winter if it should be necessary to check his sputum for antibiotic sensitivity he should attend the hospital laboratory to provide a specimen, but on no account should he bring one from home in his own container.

His anxiety at the end of treatment (eight sessions in all) was reduced to 0–2 on an 8 point scale, as measured when he felt the need to use the sputum pot, whereas it had always been 8 in this situation before treatment. The change in his behaviour, whereby he no longer felt compelled to carry the sputum pot was also remarkable. This case illustrates the importance in behavioural medicine of close collaboration with medical colleagues: no progress would have been made without convincing his physician of the behavioural formulation, and gaining his agreement and cooperation with the treatment plan.

Resistant asthma

Case illustration

A 26-year-old nurse was referred because all the standard medical treatments for her condition had been used, including large doses of steroids, but she remained disabled by respiratory symptoms, such as wheezing and difficulty in breathing.

Standard psychiatric interviews revealed many complicated problems: she had mixed feelings about her nursing career and led a lonely, isolated social life. She set herself impossibly high standards at work and when she could not achieve them, attacks of asthma led to an inability to work at all. Also she suffered from very low self-esteem, and felt hopeless about her future.

Behavioural formulation

It was hypothesised that autonomic nervous system over activity brought on the asthmatic attacks. This over activity in turn was caused by situations where she felt she had no control, which often happened at her work. The more she attempted to succeed at work and still failed, the more depressed she become. In this way a downwards spiral of ever decreasing performance ensued. Now that real handicap was caused by the symptoms, she had been told by her physician she would have to give up nursing altogether, and at the point of entry to treatment her main activity and role was that of 'a patient' (see Fig. 13.2).

Treatment

The treatment began by attempting to enable her to assess her problems realistically, and this included coping with the limitations imposed on her life by the asthma. Keeping a *diary* of attacks and noting stressful events, was helpful in pointing this out to her, and she eventually decided to leave nursing and obtained work as a GP's receptionist which produced some improvement. She also benefitted from *assertiveness training* in which, she was asked to assess the way she thought about herself, and to write down these thoughts. She wrote:

I'm a useless person, because I can't cope with nursing.

Asthma and its treatment have made me overweight and unattractive, now I'll never get a boyfriend.

As a result of the discussion in the next session she examined the evidence that these views were not the only way to assess her situation.

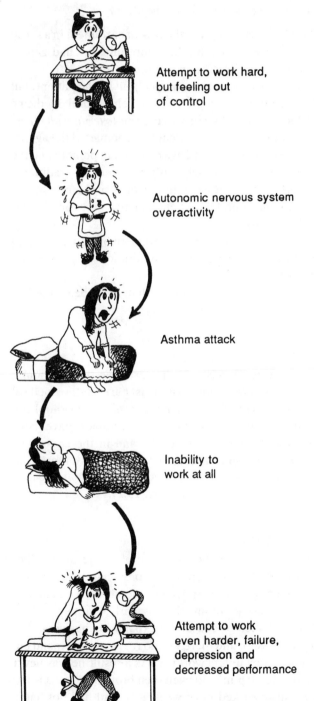

Attempt to work hard, but feeling out of control

Autonomic nervous system overactivity

Asthma attack

Inability to work at all

Attempt to work even harder, failure, depression and decreased performance

Fig. 13.2. The downwards spiral of negative thoughts.

She was not accurately assessing all the possibilities as the depressed mood was making her see only the black side. Eventually she was able to replace the above statements with:

> So you can't be a nurse – it's not the only job in the world.
> OK you are an asthmatic, but you can still get a boyfriend.

Later on in the treatment she was given the task of enrolment in a social club for graduates. She resisted joining this club until she had gained confidence from her new employment, but eventually did so.

These behavioural approaches were seen as helpful by the patient, but did not resolve her symptoms completely. In behavioural medicine patients are often helped by being taught how to *come to terms with* illness rather than bringing about a cure. The patient had completed the agreed number of 12 sessions, and so had arrived at a convenient point to end the behavioural treatment. She was subsequently referred for traditional psychotherapy, to work further on her interpersonal problems. In this case it was felt that the behavioural treatment had made it easier for this patient to seek psychotherapy.

Outcome measures showed significant improvement on depression and anxiety rating after behavioural treatment, in addition to marked improvement in lung function tests.

For details of other behavioural techniques that have been used in controlling asthma see Johnston (1984).

Hypertension

The management of hypertension is a further example of behavioural medicine. The blood pressure is monitored as part of the medical treatment, and medication is prescribed in many cases. Behavioural and cognitive factors which include relaxation and feedback have been recommended (Patel, Marmot & Terry, 1981), and in the case to be described relaxation was used, in combination with cognitive therapy to bring about changes in life-style.

Case illustration

A 50-year-old man was living a totally impossible life-style. He had moderately high blood pressure, and complained of severe palpitations for which no remedy could be discovered. The physician who referred him mentioned that the patient lived 'under considerable stress, and had an impossible life-style'. The patient said that his work meant everything to him and he was determined to constantly expand his business. The business was already successful, and there was no real need to expand but he claimed never to be happy unless working. As a result he was never home from work before 10.00 p.m. and even then brought home a brief-case full of work. He also worked most weekends, and had not had a proper holiday for many years. Because of this work pattern he had very little time to devote to his wife and two young children. The difficulties had reached a crisis shortly before he was referred, because he had started an affair with a young girl at work. He was now plagued with guilt because he felt he had let down his wife and family, and was under pressure from his girlfriend to leave his wife and make a commitment to *her*. Not surprisingly his blood pressure had risen, and his palpitations had become worse.

Behavioural formulation

Jim was on a treadmill of his own making, similar to the patient described in chapter 11, whereby his pattern of behaviour was being rewarded because work had become the only thing in life which was reinforcing. In his early days in business it had been a struggle to succeed, but this struggle was rewarded by financial success. He no longer needed the money, but the earning of money made him feel powerful, and hence continued to be rewarded. As his whole environment became work-oriented, he neglected his family more and more, and not surprisingly started an affair *at work*. The strain of this life-style was related to his hypertension and palpitations.

Treatment

The first problem to tackle in treatment was to enable the patient to keep the necessary appointments, because he could not cope with being away from his work: 'I'm losing money every hour that I spend here, I just can't stand the thought of that'.

After two failed attendances he did turn up for his appointment out of despair because he could no longer cope. A **treatment contract** was made with him that if he failed to attend he would write a cheque for £100 payable to the political party in opposition to that which he supported, for each missed appointment. This sum was agreed with the patient as an amount that he both could afford and was commensurate with the amount he might earn at work in the same period of time.

Next his work pattern was carefully discussed and it was put to him that he was on a treadmill of his own making. Work had become the only reinforcing thing in his life, and he had over the years lost interest in his former hobbies, and also lost pleasure in being with his family.

He knew about nothing else except his work, and admitted he had become a rather boring person. On the other hand he realised that work gave him a 'high', there was nothing else quite like it and he was very successful at making money. He rationalised this by saying that his children benefitted from this as the money paid for their education, and bought them other things that they enjoyed.

After our first session he announced that he had taken a holiday at last 'but it had been no good, I just couldn't relax'. On further questioning it turned out that on this 'holiday' he had taken with him his portable telephone, his portable tape recorder and fax machine, and had been in daily contact with his office! His long-suffering wife had taken the children off on day trips so as not to bother him.

The patient himself realised his 'holiday' was a sham, but it was too difficult to cut himself off from work altogether. He also agreed that he was on a treadmill but could not see how to get off. As a homework task he agreed to make a list of 'things I used to enjoy but no longer have time for', and these included:

> Going fishing with my children.
> Playing model trains with my children.
> Watching soaps on TV with my wife.
> Playing tennis.

Of these items he agreed to try to play tennis again straight away. On the next session it turned out he had hired a tennis coach to improve his game. It was pointed out that he had defeated the object of the exercise as he was learning to play *competitively*.

He then agreed that he had to make a major change in the working week, and after discussion agreed to come home no later than 6.00 p.m. each evening, and *not* to bring a briefcase or contact work in any way. He did achieve this goal, and used the time to be with his children who could not believe their luck. He then agreed not to work at all at the weekends, and if he played tennis he had to try not to win: something he found very difficult. He then went off on a proper family holiday, in which the only way he 'cheated ' was to pack a business magazine, which he subsequently threw away. It was hardly surprising that in this atmosphere the relationship with his wife improved, and the interest in his girlfriend waned.

At the end of the agreed 6 sessions he reported no trouble from palpitations, and his blood pressure was completely controlled with antihypertensive medication. In addition his anxiety and depression ratings had improved, reflecting his clinical improvement.

Diabetes related to overeating

Case illustration

A 40-year-old man with moderate obesity had been discovered to have diabetes on routine screening. His physician had referred him because the patient could not cooperate with the medical treatment regime which involved keeping to a strict diet. The patient was a self-made businessman whose great delight was going to expensive restaurants with his wife and ordering a large meal accompanied by the best wines. After his assessment session for behaviour therapy it was suggested to him that he might have to stop going to restaurants, to which he retorted: 'you must be joking, it's my main pleasure in life, I'd rather die.'

During the assessment he came across as a Falstaff-like character who enjoyed life to the full. The discovery of the diabetes was a great blow to him, because he thought it would reduce his life-span and somehow 'cheat' him out of the enjoyment of life that he considered he had earned by dint of his own efforts. He talked with pride about how he had built up the business from nothing, and how he hoped to pass it on to his children.

Behavioural formulation

Eating and drinking well were seen as rewards which the patient could not deny himself despite the knowledge that it was going to kill him. He understood perfectly the dietary implications of his diabetes, but could not overcome the established pattern of eating.

Treatment

The first behavioural task was to keep a *dietary diary* and also to *record* his weight each week on a graph. On reviewing this with him, it was clear that he ate too many carbohydrate containing foods throughout the day, and this was causing his weight problem and contributing to the diabetes. He was especially keen on extravagant foods such as caviar and lobster, and it was pointed out to him that he could eat these if he avoided the potatoes in the main meal and had fruit instead of sweet pastries for dessert. The problem of wine was resolved by asking him to find out about sugar-free wine which is suitable for diabetic consumption, and as this turned out to be very expensive he could feel he was still indulging himself.

Using this approach he managed to loose a few pounds but then went on a luxury cruise, and put the weight back on again. At this point the cognitive approach of **covert sensitisation** was used: he was asked to think of an aversive image before booking a meal in an expensive restaurant. This image was that of himself having a stroke in a restaurant after eating a large meal. He was to picture himself collapsed at the table, choking in his own vomit. He would imagine that an ambulance had been called and his wife was distraught with the sight of him. He would elaborate this imaginary scene to the utmost, and include scenes in which he was paralysed and confined to a wheelchair. As a homework task he had to write down a description of the aversive imagery and attach one copy to the front of his favourite restaurant guide and another to the front of the refrigerator. Using these techniques he was able to reduce some weight and bring the diabetes under control at the end of 10 sessions. As he put it in his own words 'I can't enjoy life much from a wheelchair'.

Epilepsy

Epilepsy is caused by an abnormal electrical activity of the brain, but it is another example of a disorder with multifactorial causation. Feldman &

Norman, (1976) described how patients can be taught to recognise the association between certain stressful stimuli and the seizure. In their work videotapes were played back to patients to help them confront situations that were stressful, and a similar confrontation technique was used in the case described below but without the use of videotapes.

Case illustration

Bill was a 20-year-old university student whose *grand mal* attacks were only partially controlled by medication. He was finding some difficulties with his studies and tended to be preoccupied with obsessive thoughts of a philosophical kind such as 'what are we all doing here, what is the meaning of life', but he had no other obsessional features. He complained of feeling tired a great deal of the time, but would often stay up late at student parties or other social activities.

Treatment

Self-monitoring was carried out in which he noted stressful events, preoccupation with obsessional thinking, and frequency of fits. After three weeks a pattern emerged in which it was clear that late nights increased the likelihood of having fits. Some slight improvement was achieved when Bill altered his life-style but this improvement was not impressive, and had social disadvantages: he could not live the normal life of a university student.

At the third session a pattern of increased preoccupation with philosophical-doubting thoughts was noted prior to fits. On talking about this with Bill, he related this to his extremely religious upbringing as a child and talked with great anger about this:

BILL: I think this was when my troubles started. I was terrified into believing in God and made to feel guilty if I questioned anything the priest said.
THERAPIST: Do you still feel angry with anyone about this?
BILL: My parents. They said if I prayed enough the fits would stop, and as a child I believed them of course. I recognise anger welling up in me now just before I get the fit.

The *formulation* at this point was that pent up angry feelings could be the trigger for a fit. If he was *exposed* to these feelings when he was relaxed and unlikely to have a fit, habituation would occur, and the emotional power of the feelings would diminish.

Treatment then focused on six sessions in which Bill was first of all given brief relaxation exercises (as described in the Appendix 1), then asked to 'think angry thoughts about your parents' for 20 to 30 minutes. He was able to this very successfully, and at the end of these sessions the frequency of fits was greatly diminished.

Cognitive-behavioural treatment for epilepsy was a useful component of the overall management of the case, but the use of these techniques is still in its infancy, and controlled trials with long-term outcome are lacking. Nevertheless this case shows how *cognitive-behavioural principles* can be applied to a medical condition where at first sight they may seem to have no role.

Abdominal pain

Case illustration

Jill was seen initially on a home visit at the request of her GP. She was lying in bed moaning saying, 'I've never been so bad, you have got to give me some tablets to help, I don't want my husband to lose his job but I can't cope without him here all the time.' Then she described a back pain that her GP knew all about, and that had been exhaustively investigated despite which no organic cause could be found. When this was pointed out to her she then described an abdominal pain, again for which no organic cause could be discovered. Her husband was in danger of loosing his job because he frequently took time off work to be with his wife: even if he managed to get to work on time she telephoned him at work and made him return home in his lunch hour. She also called out her GP several times each week because of back or abdominal pain, and always claimed to be too ill to go to his surgery. The GP had been initially sympathetic but was rapidly loosing patience with her, as each time she requested another kind of medication or referral to another specialist.

Illness behaviour can be defined as seeking attention by presenting symptoms of illness, which cannot be explained medically. In this case Jill's dependence on her husband is clear, and this dependence had worsened recently after her mother died. She had learnt how to gain her husband's attention by showing symptoms of backache or abdominal pain, and so the focus of treatment had to involve working with Jill's husband, who said: 'But I can't just go back to work and leave her to scream, what will the neighbours say?'

It was difficult to understand how he had put up with her behaviour for so long, but it is often the case that spouses of patients with illness behaviour are often caught in the trap of providing reassurance to their loved one. This is a pattern that has to be broken, and was done so in this case by behavioural exchange therapy as described in chapter 8. This began with a session talking about what each of them expected from the other, and how this could be achieved. Jill's husband expected to be able to get to work on time, and not to be called home in his lunch hour. Jill herself wanted a show of affection from her husband, but as long as this was provided once a day the timing of it was not crucial to her. It was therefore agreed that Jill's husband would talk to her for one hour in the evening, and during this time would give her his undivided attention. Jill's part of the bargain would be that she would not delay his going to work, nor would she telephone him to call him home at lunch time.

Another key person in the treatment contract was her GP who agreed to see Jill in future by appointment only, at not more than an agreed frequency which was gradually extended in time so that in six months Jill was only visiting him once a month, a service he was perfectly happy to provide. In order for Jill to travel to the GP's surgery her husband had to take her in the car after work, as she could not travel alone. The next stage was a course of *graduated exposure* using her husband as co-therapist along the lines described in chapter 3. He initially took her to the corner shop until her fear in that situation decreased, and then gradually further afield until she could cope with public transport and go anywhere she wished to alone. As she gained in independence and her confidence improved, Jill was able to obtain a voluntary job, thus ending once and for all her 'career' as a patient.

The psychological aspects of pain in general covers a large field, much of which is reviewed by Merskey (1984).

Vomiting fear

Case illustration

Doreen had been investigated by numerous gastroenterologists and nothing organic had been found. She had been told she had a 'sensitive stomach' and this was the cause of her constant nausea and fear that she might vomit. The eventual psychiatric referral brought out a very long history of a fear of *other people* being sick and avoidance of any situation where she might possibly see people vomiting. She avoided parties, restaurants, cinemas, theatres and any street where there was a public house, in case she encountered drunks because they might vomit. The investigations for stomach disorder were stopped when the patient was persuaded that she was seeking treatment that was bound to fail, as there was no stomach disorder. The illness behaviour was manifest, because it was more acceptable for this patient to have a medical label, rather than a psychiatric one.

Treatment

Treatment was started by devising a programme for her to re-expose to the avoided situations. She agreed to walk down streets with public houses at times when drunks could be expected to be on the streets. This was not successful as she did not, in fact, encounter anyone vomiting. The fear remained that she *might* encounter a vomiting drunk person, and so avoidance continued. Next she was asked to concoct a recipe for 'vomit' using chopped vegetables and tins of pea soup. Her homework task was to make this substance and to pour it out into the lavatory pan while imagining it to be vomit. This produced only a slight reduction in fear of *actual* vomit, as one of the main features of actual vomit is it's unpredictability of appearance: 'you never really know when you or somebody else is going to be sick'.

Finally, success was achieved by using a specially prepared videotape of a doctor interviewing an actor pretending to feel sick and then apparently being sick. This five minute videotape was made into a loop whereby it repeated until it lasted for one hour. This provided very realistic exposure to the feared situation that the patient found most helpful. After she had played the tape daily for three weeks, she was able to walk outside public houses, and went to restaurants with her husband for the first time in 20 years.

Insomnia

It has been said that preoccupation with obtaining the right amount and quality of sleep in our time in history, has replaced the fashionable preoccupation with bowel action from the Victorian era. Certainly a great deal has been written on the psychological aspects of insomnia (e.g. Borkovec, 1982).

Assessment is crucially important if treatment is to be effective. Enquiries should be made of the pattern of sleep onset, the use of stimulant drugs (including tea and coffee) and the use of alcohol, and of sleeping tablets. Keeping diary records of these factors is very useful and may itself be therapeutic.

Case illustration

A patient was referred from a physician for behavioural treatment for *pain* in her neck, for which no organic reason could be discovered. When a full history had been taken, she disclosed that the pain was not her main concern, but she was worried about inadequate sleep at night. She claimed that she could not get off to sleep unless she took a sleeping tablet (20 mg temazepam), and she was sure that her performance at work was poor on the days when her sleep had been unsatisfactory the night before. She worked as a salesperson on commission, was enthusiastic about her job, and pushed herself hard. The reason she lay awake at night was *not* due to the pain in her neck, which had gone after a course of physiotherapy. It was clear that she would go to bed and worry about not sleeping, and this in turn would reduce the likelihood of her getting to sleep.

Treatment

The patient was asked to keep a diary of the time she went to bed, and the following day to record the time she thought she actually went to sleep.

She was also to record the use of any medication, alcohol, tea or coffee. In addition, she recorded any stressful event or worry that she might have had at the time.

She was asked to read a self-help book: *Sleep* by I. M. Oswald (1966), and to carry out the advice therein, to avoid tea or coffee after 6.00 p.m., and to try going to bed at the same regular time, and to avoid 'catnaps' during the day. In addition, she was given the taped relaxation practice, as described in the Appendix 1.

These simple measures to improve 'sleep hygiene' are often dramatically effective, and so are worth trying first. However, if this alone does not work, as in the above case, two further techniques can be tried: **paradoxical intention** and *stimulus control*.

Paradoxical intention

This patient lay in bed at night worrying about the consequences of not getting enough sleep. This worry itself prevented her going to sleep. Using the paradoxical technique she was asked to prevent herself going to sleep as much as possible. She was told, 'Try *not* to go to sleep for as long as you can. Some experiments on sleep deprivation show that people feel *better* for less sleep. Let us see if this can work for you'.

Stimulus control

This technique involves consideration of the conditioning factors that may operate to induce sleep. The theory is that if you are surrounded by familiar 'safe' objects you are more likely to associate them with sleep, and therefore may actually go to sleep. Beds and bedrooms should have sleep associations, but may have many other associations too. If bed is where you write your letters and watch TV, then it may acquire the wrong stimulus associations.

The patient described above did her accounts in bed, and when this was pointed out she arranged to read a woman's magazine instead. She deliberately chose the magazine because of its bland slightly boring content. This switch in behaviour produced an improvement in sleep.

The general problem of insomnia, and the role of medication are discussed in detail by Oswald (1984).

Summary

· Behavioural medicine is the application of behavioural and cognitive therapy to medicine. It includes the management of conditions subsumed under psychosomatic medicine, hypochondriasis and illness behaviour.

· A cognitive model is described, which suggests that thoughts of illness in patients with hypochondriasis are similar to the obsessional ideas of patients with obsessive-compulsive disorder.

- From the model a treatment is derived which involves education, banning medical reassurance, cognitive restructuring and behavioural testing.
- In behavioural medicine meaningful liaison with medical colleagues is crucial.
- Dietary and life-style factors are crucial in many cases.
- Self-monitoring is valuable along with standard cognitive and behavioural approaches, such as the setting of homework tasks.
- In many cases in behavioural medicine, cure is not possible, but small symptomatic improvement can often bring about large changes in the quality of life.

14 Medication

Whatever you do don't give me any more of those useless pills.

Can't you give me some pills to take that will make me feel better, instead of this difficult (behaviour) therapy.

These contradictory remarks made by our patients exemplify some of the problems. Other problems surround fashions in medical prescribing habits as shown in Fig. 14.1.

Patients differ in their *expectations* of both medication and behaviour therapy. It is therefore not surprising that some regimes will suit some patients but not others. The role of medication in behavioural and cognitive therapy will be discussed under 5 headings:

1   Exposure therapy and benzodiazepines.
2   Exposure therapy and tricyclic medication.
3   Exposure therapy and beta-blockers.
4   The treatment of obsessive-compulsive disorder and antidepressant medication.

Fig. 14.1. Prescribing patterns vary with the fashion.

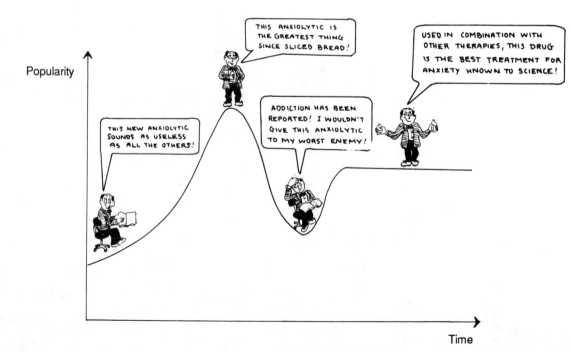

5   Cognitive therapy of depression and antidepressant medication.

Exposure therapy and benzodiazepines

A 35-year-old woman with typical features of agoraphobia said 'Whatever else you do I am not taking any more of those useless pills. My doctor started me off on Librium, then he changed it to Valium, then I was drowsy all day so I was switched to Ativan. They say on TV that these pills are addictive so now I suppose I'm a drug addict as well as still being completely housebound.'

The theoretical outcomes of combining behaviour therapy and benzodiazepines have been discussed by Wardle (1990). They may be *mutually beneficial*, for example by inducing the ideal conditions for maximal habituation or extinction, by reducing the patient's arousal levels. They might also help by reducing the unpleasantness of exposure therapy. On the other hand there may be *harmful effects* which could operate by the mechanism of state-dependant learning effects, and this could prevent generalisation of new learning from the drug state to the non-drug state. State-dependant learning occurs when learning takes place under the influence of a drug, and this learning does not transfer to the non-drug state. This is known to occur in a number of drugs including alcohol. Gray (1987) has suggested that benzodiazepines might impair the effectiveness of behaviour therapy by attenuating the development of behavioural tolerance to stress.

Giving medication to patients can have many effects apart from these purely pharmacological ones. The so called '**attribution effect**' may be important. This is where the patient may carry out an exposure exercise after taking a particular medication, saying that they do so *because* of the drug. The effect of the drug may have been to boost the patient's confidence through a psychological mechanism, although the patient himself attributes this to a pharmacological one. Other truly pharmacological effects are **tolerance** and withdrawal. Tolerance means that increasingly larger amounts of medication have to be given to produce the same effect, and is a very real danger with the benzodiazepine group of drugs. Withdrawal effects occur with the same group of drugs, and withdrawal effects are the pharmacological effects of stopping the drug. One of the most important of these is that panic attacks can be caused: clearly of great clinical relevance given that this is very often the clinical condition which it sought to treat.

The studies carried out in patients show contradictory findings, but there is tentative evidence that behavioural treatment is associated with lower levels of anxiety during exposure in patients taking anxiolytics.

In a controlled study of 60 patients who have agoraphobia with panic attacks or panic disorder, some patients were given alprazolam in a four-month combined drug and behavioural group treatment programme.

One of the major findings was that the efficacy of alprazolam and behavioural therapy in the short-term treatment of panic appeared to be maintained during long-term alprazolam maintenance. Also, sustained clinical improvements were observed in many patients who decreased or discontinued alprazolam (Nagy *et al.*, 1989).

Diazepam given in moderate doses just before exposure made no difference to the outcome, but given in regular doses was better than propranalol (Noyes *et al.*, 1984). Therapists have stated that failure to habituate to exposure often seems related to ingestion of large amounts of benzodiazepines or alcohol (Marks & O'Sullivan, 1988). Despite this it is our experience that *some* cases are helped to overcome avoidance by small doses of diazepam:

Case illustration

'I will never get on that underground train unless I can take 5 mg of Valium just before', stated a 24-year-old woman who had developed fears of travelling on the underground two years earlier for no apparent reason. She worked in the City of London and had to use this mode of transport despite the discomfort it caused her every day. She had no avoidance as long as she took the Valium tablet and she had considered taking the tablet for ever until put under pressure by her own doctor to stop them.

Assessment

The tablet may have a direct anxiolytic effect which makes it easier to cope with the feared situation. In addition there is a strong psychological effect: each time she swallows it she expects to feel better and this expectation is reinforced each time she takes it and *does* feel better. The problem of treatment is that if she ventures into the feared situation without medication she would expect to feel worse.

Treatment

The patient was motivated to come off medication because of her fear of remaining on it. She was persuaded to undergo self-exposure homework exercises along the lines described in chapter 5, but would only agree to do so with some medication. The dose was therefore reduced, initially to 2 mg for one week, then 1 mg for one week, so that eventually she was able to travel without taking any medication. She still insisted on *carrying* a small supply of 1 mg tablets in her handbag, but had not actually taken any of these when seen at follow-up one year later.

One could possibly explain the mechanism of medication in terms of safety signal theory (Gray, 1987). This theory implies that the small amount of medication had become conditioned to 'safety' and so the tablets were no longer necessary for any pharmacological action, although they originally did have.

Exposure therapy and tricyclic medication

As far back as 1964, the New York psychiatrist Klein suggested that imipramine might lower anticipatory anxiety in agoraphobia. Zitrin, Klein & Woerner (1980) reported that imipramine was superior to placebo in both agoraphobic and 'mixed phobic' groups, although not in 'simple phobics'. In that study, supportive psychotherapy and systematic desensitisation were also compared in patients receiving either drug or placebo. The combination of supportive psychotherapy plus imipramine was slightly superior to the combination of desensitisation in fantasy plus imipramine. As discussed in chapter 1, we now consider desensitisation in fantasy to be a very weak treatment. Another problem that has made interpretation difficult for this and similar studies, is that patients may obtain self-exposure in an uncontrolled way, because it becomes known that 'self-exposure makes you better' when they attend a phobia clinic. There have been 10 subsequent studies of imipramine, making this the most widely studied drug. These are all reviewed by Marks & O'Sullivan (1988) who point out that there have been eight studies in which imipramine was better than placebo in agoraphobia/panic disorder. Marks & O'Sullivan conclude that imipramine usually yields a short term reduction in many agoraphobic symptoms but the effect is broad-spectrum and non-specific. The size of the drug effect is unclear, and it has a delayed onset as would be expected. Exposure therapy facilitates the effect of imipramine, but it could also be that imipramine facilitates the effect of exposure.

In order to pursue this question Telch *et al.* (1985) randomly assigned 37 severely disabled agoraphobic patients to:

1   A group receiving imipramine and no exposure.
2   A group receiving imipramine *plus* exposure.
3   A placebo plus exposure group.

To provide a more stringent test of the pharmacological effects of imipramine independent of exposure to phobic stimuli, patients in group 1 received anti-exposure instructions during the first eight weeks of therapy. At eight weeks the group receiving imipramine combined with exposure therapy showed more improvement than the other two groups, and was the only group to show a reduction in panic attacks. This favourable response to the combined use of imipramine and exposure is consistent with the findings of Zitrin *et al.* (1980), but discrepant with that of Marks *et al.* (1983) who found no synergistic effect.

In clinical practice there probably is a role for combining exposure therapy with imipramine in cases where the patient lacks confidence to venture into the feared situation and suffers from panic attacks, bearing in mind that a substantial number of patients are fearful of medication, and many cannot tolerate the drug's side effects. Nevertheless, some cases do benefit, as illustrated:

> The ideas I have read about in that book you gave me (*Living With Fear*, by I. M. Marks) are all very well but I can never get into the supermarket because of the state I get into outside. I tremble, shake and sweat so much I just have to go home in the end, even though I know I should go inside like it says in the book.

This patient was then put on imipramine starting with 25 mg daily for one week, and increasing by 25 mg increments each week until she was taking 75 mg at the end of the third week. She then found that the panic attacks were less severe and she could continue with the kind of self exposure programme fully described in chapter 5. She remained on 75 mg imipramine for a three-month period, after which the drug was withdrawn. She remained free of phobic symptoms at one year follow-up.

There have been studies of other antidepressant drugs, but the information is too sparse to come to any definite conclusions about their value in combination with exposure therapy.

Exposure therapy and beta-blockers

There are conflicting studies on the research in this area. For instance Ullrich *et al*. (1975) found beta-blockers were superior to placebo when given along with exposure therapy, but Noyes *et al*. (1984) found them to be inferior to diazepam. Beta-blockers in moderate doses have no central effects on the nervous system, so the mode of action depends on peripheral blockade of the sympathetically mediated mechanisms underlying the symptom. As pointed out in chapter 11, bodily symptoms may reinforce anxiety, and a vicious cycle can be set up. Therefore, in patients in whom *tremor*, *palpitations* or *diarrhoea* are the major symptoms, beta-blockers can have an important role in combination with the cognitive therapy of anxiety states. As with all medication, treatment has to be weighed against side-effects, which are relatively few with this class of drug, but in some patients this can include faintness, which the patient may find unbearable. The dosage of medication has to be tailored to the individual patient, for example with propranalol it is often commenced at 10 mg and increased gradually to 120 mg daily.

The treatment of obsessive-compulsive disorder and antidepressant medication

Clomipramine is the only drug to have been extensively studied in the treatment of obsessive-compulsive disorder. From the earliest reports (Lopez-Ibor, 1966) to the most recent (Marks *et al*., 1988) there have been a large number of studies, most of which show that clomipramine reduced obsessional symptoms, in addition to reducing anxiety and depression. It is still debatable as to whether the drug has a *specific* anti-obsessional effect: Marks *et al.*, (1988) argue that *where clomipramine had an effect, improvement was not only in obsessive-compulsive symptoms but also on depression, anxiety and any other symptoms being measured, and moreover there was no evidence that the obsessive-compulsive symptoms remitted first before any other symptoms that were present.* They also point out that relapse is frequent within months of stopping the drug, and long-term benefits from medication were absent in two 2-year follow-up studies after clomipramine (Mawson, Marks & Ramm, 1982; Kasvikis & Marks, 1988). The latter study also suggests that rituals and mood were relatively independent variables.

Those who argue for a specific anti-obsessional effect for clomipramine point out that it is a relatively selective and potent inhibitor of active serotonin uptake in the brain. Mavissakalian *et al.*, (1985) found that clomipramine was *equally* effective in high and low depressed patients with obsessive-compulsive disorder, which along with studies carried out in children (Leonard *et al.*, 1988) makes the case for a specific anti-obsessional effect. Further suggestion for a specific effect comes from the study of Stern *et al.*, (1980) in which plasma concentration of clomipramine and its primary metabolite N-desmethylclomipramine were measured: plasma clomipramine concentration was related to outcome of *rituals* while the metabolite concentration was related to outcome of *depression*.

The *specific serotonin re-uptake blockers* have also been studied in obsessive-compulsive disorder. Contradictory findings resulted with zimelidine, but this drug has now been withdrawn. Price *et al.* (1987) found significant improvement in a single blind placebo controlled study of fluvoxamine. Another selective serotonin re-uptake inhibitor, fluoxetine, has been effective in a single blind trial (Turner *et al.*, 1985), and further controlled trials are awaited.

The task of investigating the relationship between clomipramine's serotonergic effect and its effect in obsessive-compulsive disorder was carried out in a unique way by Benkelfat *et al.*, (1989). They gave metergoline, a serotonin receptor antagonist, and placebo to 10 patients in a double blind crossover study. Patients were all already on clomipramine on a long-term basis with a 40 per cent lessening of symptoms. They responded to four days of metergoline therapy with significantly *greater* obsessive-compulsive disorder symptoms, supporting the specific serotonergic hypothesis for the action of clomipramine.

Case illustration of value of clomipramine

Charles was a 45-year-old man preoccupied with meticulous checking rituals. Every time he left the house he was compelled to check that he had locked the doors and windows, following a long procedure that took about two hours. He had all the classical features of obsessive-compulsive disorder as described in chapter 4, and was a very suitable case for graduated exposure with response prevention. However, he refused to come into hospital, and was even reluctant to allow a therapist to visit him at home. He was, therefore given instructions to carry out exposure plus *self-imposed* response prevention in combination with clomipramine. The dose was 25 mg at night for one week, then 50 mg at night for one week, followed by 75 mg, which continued for a further month. He reported that the tablets seemed to make it easier to carry out the exposure and self-imposed response prevention. The dose was later on gradually increased to 200 mg which seemed to produce an even greater benefit, in that he was able to reduce the checking rituals so that it only took him 15 minutes before he could leave his home.

When seen for follow-up at six months and one year, the improvement had been maintained, but he reported a well known side-effect: anorgasmia (he was unable to ejaculate). It can be seen as a tribute to the drug that he was prepared to endure this side-effect, rather than come off the medication at this stage saying: 'sex is one thing, but those rituals totally controlled my life. Given the choice I would prefer to carry on with the tablets.'

This case illustrates where clomipramine seemed helpful, despite having side-effects. However, cases could also be cited where the side effects, in particular constipation and dry mouth, have been so severe that the patient insisted in being taken off the medication. Often patients with obsessive-compulsive disorder are less able to cope with medication and with side-effects, because the disorder itself makes them check for any possible effect of the drug.

Cognitive therapy of depression and antidepressant medication

It is generally recommended that antidepressant medication is of value in those cases of depression where biological symptoms (sleep and appetite disturbance) predominate. However, the current view of depression is that it represents a spectrum of disorders with those cases with predominantly biological symptoms at one end, those with mainly psychological symptoms at the other but *most* cases falling somewhere in between. It follows that many cases should be amenable to a *combination* of cognitive therapy and antidepressant medication. One difficulty is that we cannot yet specify from research data *which* cases will be most suitable for this combined approach, although some guidelines may be given. It is likely that medication *plus* cognitive therapy are indicated in the following:

> Evidence for biological symptoms (e.g. weight and sleep disturbance) *in addition* to clear cognitive features.

Resistant depression with chronic history of short term response to therapy alone, where all the usual methods including lithium therapy have been tried.

Medication alone has not succeeded.

Cognitive therapy alone has not succeeded.

Case illustration of treatment of resistant depression

A 55-year-old married woman with no children complained of depression which had troubled her for eight years. She had a large number of somatic complaints which included: mucous discharging from her eyes, intermittent abdominal pain, joint pain in hands and feet and chronic constipation. She could not sleep, despite taking sleeping tablets, her appetite was poor, and she had lost weight. The somatic symptoms were worse when she was depressed.

She had been referred after intensive investigation by her physician, who had not been able to uncover any cause for her symptoms apart from suspecting 'an underlying depressive illness'. On assessment, there did not appear to be any precipitating stress for her depression, except that she was finding it hard to come to terms with the fact that she was getting older, and because of some arthritis could no longer be as active as she would wish.

In the past she had been treated with three different kinds of antidepressant medication, but each had been stopped because of side-effects. She was not convinced that medication of any kind could help her, was reluctant to change her current medication which consisted of: analgesic tablets for arthritis, benzodiazepine sleeping tablets at double the recommended dose, benzodiazepine tranquilliser taken three times each day, and a daily laxative each morning.

Treatment

After the assessment had been completed the next step was to convince the patient that the depression she was suffering from was related to the bulk of her complaints, and that this might be amenable to the combined approach of cognitive therapy and antidepressant medication. It was pointed out that she had not really tested the hypothesis about whether antidepressant tablets could help because she had not taken them for long enough in the past, and those she was taking currently were tranquillisers *not* antidepressants. Instead of having the view 'no doctors can help me', she was gradually persuaded that it might be useful to try the experiment to test the hypothesis that a different treatment might work.

The next step was to rationalise her current medication, and to do this it was necessary to find out her beliefs about tablets, and where she had obtained these ideas. Part of her belief was folklore 'you have to have a bowel action each morning after breakfast, or else you must take a laxative'. Part of her ideas come from a friend 'unless she takes her Valium (diazepam) regularly she becomes very tense, I reckon I ought to do the same'. Some information was from articles in a woman's magazine warning against antidepressant medication, claiming that it causes weight gain, constipation and drowsiness. It was then possible to dispute the evidence for these statements pointing out also where truths had been mixed in with fictions, for example many antidepressants *can* cause constipation but in her case many other factors may be to blame such as her poor diet, and also her incorrect assumption about the need to have a daily bowel action.

The next step was to persuade her to reduce the existing medication, and she eventually saw the logic of this beginning by stopping the daily laxative. She then realised that the daily tranquilliser might be making her drowsy, so she decided to stop that.

After two weeks the increasing weight loss was giving cause for concern, and so she agreed to start the experiment using imipramine, a tricyclic antidepressant. She was told to *expect* side-effects such as constipation and dry mouth, but instead of letting her persuade herself 'this proves the tablets are harmful' she was able to say to herself 'this is just what the doctor predicted would happen, as that is the case, it could be that he is also right in saying they might help me'. She was also given information about the medication to read as a homework exercise, (pp. 233–8 from *Living with Fear* by I. M. Marks).

After three weeks on medication there was a slight improvement in appetite, and the focus of the next six sessions switched to cognitive factors while the dose of medication was gradually built up. She was asked to record negative thoughts as outlined in chapter 12 and these formed the basis for discussion in the sessions. It was clear that she dwelt on her physical disability (arthritis) and had gradually stopped most of her former activities and interests. For example, she said 'I can't belong to the Woman's Voluntary Organisation any more because I am no use to anyone'. She was encouraged to test this by going to another meeting and it transpired that several other woman had greater problems with arthritis, but could still make a contribution. As a homework exercise she was asked to read *Coping with Depression* by I. Blackburn, and to rate herself on Beck's 21-item self-rating scale for depression which that book contains, and she scored 35 (severe depression).

During the course of cognitive therapy, medication was also reviewed, and she agreed to try to stop the sleeping tablets, and minimise the amount of analgesics she took. The analgesic contained codeine, which in addition to causing constipation is addictive. At the end of 12 weeks, during which she was seen once every two weeks she was only taking a tranquilliser once a week at most, and was on full recommended doses of imipramine. Her Beck depression score was reduced to 9, she was putting on weight, and no longer so preoccupied with physical symptoms.

This patient remained free of depression at one year follow-up, which was six months after antidepressants had been withdrawn. This resistant case shows how it can be necessary to change the patient's attitudes to medication for it to produce benefit, and this can be done by hypothesis testing with the patient's collaboration, and combined with other cognitive approaches such as the diary of negative thoughts, early in the therapy.

The place of combined cognitive and drug therapy

Many therapists would limit cognitive therapy to those cases where medication cannot be used for some reason, mainly because cognitive therapy is more time-consuming than medication. However, some recent studies suggest that cognitive therapy may prevent the rate of relapse after drug therapy, and this could be a good reason for the use of a combined approach (Hollon *et al.*, 1984; Simons *et al.*, 1986; Blackburn, Funson & Bishop, 1986). These findings have yet to be replicated in larger samples, but if this is done the combined approach may well have a major role in future, as one of the enduring problems with depression is to prevent relapse.

A full description of current research in this area would be out of place in this volume, but mention of the NIMH treatment of depression study is warranted at this point (Elkin *et al.*, 1989). This large study compared interpersonal psychotherapy, cognitive behaviour therapy, imipramine plus standard clinical management, and placebo plus standard clinical management. There was a consistent ordering of treatment effects at the end of the 16-week study, with imipramine plus standard clinical management doing best and placebo plus clinical management the worst, with the two psychotherapies in between but generally closer to imipramine plus clinical management. The two psychological treatments have never before been compared within the same study, but the general lack of differences in outcome between them is consistent with much in the psychotherapy literature. Future publications from the same team promise to consider the role of psychological therapies in maintenance of improvement, and in prevention of relapse. This study should be borne in mind in relation to cognitive therapy for depression (chapter 12), as it suggests that cognitive therapy is no better than interpersonal therapy.

Summary

- The benzodiazepine group of drugs have a therapeutic role in combination with exposure in some patients.
- The beneficial effects of benzodiazepines are discussed in relation to helping habituation to feared stimuli, reducing arousal and making the treatment more pleasant.

- The harmful effects of benzodiazepines can include tolerance, state-dependant learning and withdrawal problems.
- There is a role for the combination of exposure therapy and imipramine in some cases of agoraphobia, and in panic disorder, especially where pure behavioural/cognitive methods have not been successful.
- Beta-blocker drugs may be helpful combined with exposure therapy for particular anxiety symptoms, but findings are contradictory.
- Clomipramine has been advocated in obsessive-compulsive disorder, combined with exposure and response prevention. There is still no consensus about the exact effect of this drug, many pointing out that the drug is not that effective in the long term.
- The combination of cognitive therapy and antidepressant medication, in the treatment of depression may prove especially useful in preventing relapse of depressive illness.

15 Conclusion

We would like to conclude this book with some speculations on the future of behavioural and cognitive psychotherapy, in addition to some ideas on preventative treatment.

'When ten years ago I found myself turning away hundreds of patients from treatment by placing them on a waiting list receding into infinity, I was led to search for ways of treating neurotic patients more economically' (Marks, 1981). This comment anticipated and accurately predicted the development of the non-medical role in therapy, which proceeds apace. Nurse-therapists were shown to be as effective as other therapists (Marks, Connolly & Philpott, 1977) and it is likely that more therapy in future will be carried out in this way. Medical students proved to be effective behaviour therapists, but of course required careful supervision, treating prudently selected and straightforward cases of phobic disorder (Stern, 1975). It is likely that more therapy may be carried out by general medical practitioners in future, just as this group are now being encouraged to carry out more procedures from other specialities, for example minor surgical operations.

The cheapest form of therapy is self-therapy. In most of the chapters in this book we have referred to the use of self-help books, and it is likely that these will have an increasing role in future developments. One could envisage self-help packages being developed along behavioural/cognitive lines, which patients themselves could set up and run with minimal professional supervision, using various self-help books. Audio and video-tapes could be incorporated into self-help packages, and a number of audiotapes for self-help are already commercially available. Adequate professional supervision will always be important and a cautionary tale may be related: a self-help group was set up for a group of agoraphobic housewives, and seemed to run well for about a year. Then one of the authors contacted a member of the group to check on its progress and found all the group members had given up going out of the house altogether! They had decided to telephone each other every day, and the social contact by telephone meant they never needed to go out, which reinforced the very pathology the group had been set up to counteract.

Another way of providing cheap self-help is to use computers to administer the treatment. The original scepticism expressed about such methods has proved unfounded. Computers can be programmed to take case histories, and administer all the standard questionnaires. In addition they can provide 'intelligent feedback', that is the programme will respond to the patient's input in a manner designed to improve his future performance in a behavioural task. Much of this area remains to be tested but Ghosh (1981) has described the role of computers in the therapy of phobic disorders. The use of computer-administered cognitive/ behavioural therapy for depression has been evaluated, by randomly assigning depressed patients to computer-administered cognitive/ behavioural treatment, to therapist administered cognitive/behavioural treatment, or to a waiting list control. After treatment, and at two-month follow-up, both treatment groups improved significantly more than controls (Selmi *et al.*, 1990). One could foresee further developments of computer applications in therapy for a range of disorders.

Prevention

Prevention is better than cure. This often quoted ideal is seldom pursued in practice by those responsible for funding research, so that little is known about prevention of psychological disorders. One might speculate from social learning theories that child-rearing practices may influence the development of many of the disorders described in this book. Exposure therapy would predict that teaching your child to study spiders and encouraging their natural curiosity about the world, would be a better modelling experience than the mother who jumps on a chair whenever a small animal appears on the kitchen floor. The learning of fear is a complex area, but one aspect is the well known phenomenon of 'incubation', that is the delay between a trauma and onset of a symptom, which is described by Marks (1987). The value of this knowledge in prevention of phobias is also known to folklore: if you fall off your horse you should get on the horse again as soon as possible, if not, fear will increase and you may never ride again. In clinical practice, patients with a tendency to be agoraphobic may become phobic again if they have to remain indoors for a prolonged period of time, for example after an attack of influenza. They should be advised to venture outside as soon as their physical condition permits in order to minimise risk of a relapse of agoraphobia.

Turning to obsessive-compulsive disorder, the role of parental model-ling may be important. The authors have seen cases where children have been made to carry out rituals by their obsessional parent. Clearly treating the parent not only for their sake, but for the sake of the next generation could be very important, although the well known genetic component in obsessive-compulsive disorder cannot be discounted. This subject is reviewed by Murray & Reveley (1981).

Another area where parental influences may contribute is that of social skills deficit. The parents whose family meals consist of each partner staring at each other, or one reading the newspaper while the other does the washing up are not likely to be the best role models for the future generation. Communication skills are also most likely learnt across generations, although not necessarily from the parents to the children. Education about sex could do much to eliminate sexual anxiety in adults. We have seen a patient who thought he was homosexual for no other reason that he masturbated. He had been taught that this activity was an 'unnatural practice' and jumped to the wrong conclusion.

In addition to the above examples of the preventative value of education, there may be an increasing role in the sphere of marital discord. Stuart (1973) has developed an inventory to give to couples who attend for pre-marital counselling. The aims are to help a couple disclose aspects that may underlie their thinking about the potential marriage, and to help them formulate goals during courtship. Also, many of the techniques used in behavioural marital therapy aim to prevent trouble occurring, for example the technique of 'conflict containment', whereby the couple is helped to select issues that might be acting as conflict triggers, find the least potentially damaging means of expressing anger, and shift into problem solving, as described in chapter 8. Effective marital therapy may reduce the divorce rate, and divorce is statistically correlated with depression and with suicide. It could be argued that divorce is a liberating experience for many people who should not stay together, but behavioural marital therapy could help a couple reach just this conclusion. We do not yet have a predictive test that would tell us at the outset of therapy which marriages will succeed and which will fail.

Prevention plays a role in changing behaviour in the chronic patient, mainly in the prevention of the effects of institutionalisation. The importance of care rather than cure has already been emphasised in chapter 10.

Turning to the subject of chapter 11, the treatment of non-phobic anxiety, much has been written on **stress immunisation** or 'stress inoculation training' (Meichenbaum, 1977). Briefly, these approaches involve a discussion of stress reactions, rehearsing coping skills, and testing these skills under actual stressful conditions. Meichenbaum exposed snake-phobic volunteers to the phobic stimulus, and taught coping self-statements during this exercise. This is similar to the approaches used today for cognitive therapy of anxiety states. The concept of teaching *coping* to provide a method of dealing with future symptoms can be seen as a preventative method. However, it is too simplistic to make the analogy between this, and the prevention of a disease such as smallpox by the *inoculation* of cowpox, as described by Edward Jenner (1798) in probably the most important book ever published on prevention of disease. We do not yet have an anti-anxiety vaccine.

One of the arguments put forward in favour of cognitive therapy for depression is that it prevents the likelihood of future relapse (Paykel,

1989). Once more the model is one of the therapist as educator, teaching coping skills and leaving the patient with a package of tools to mend the 'machine' if it goes wrong using the tools (or techniques) that have been taught during therapy. Patients are taught the following steps: first specify the problem, next develop a hypothesis about what is causing the problem, then test out your hypothesis. They are then taught how to evaluate whether their hypothesis works or not and to act accordingly. The patient learns 'this worked for me in the past, the chances are it's going to work for me in the future'. A related area in which prevention may be of value is in ensuring that grief is adequately dealt with. Bereaved widows helped in this way did better at 13-month follow-up than controls (Raphael, 1977). It is also known that social factors are causative in depression: social class, numbers of children under school age, and the lack of a supportive husband (Brown & Harris, 1978). Clearly women in certain categories are at high risk from depression, and in preventative terms apart from wider social issues, the only factor that may be amenable to change might be the relationship with the husband, using some of the approaches described in chapter 8.

In chapter 13 a number of cognitive therapies for hypochondriasis were described. It was also implied that medicine might be to blame in many cases of hypochondriasis, largely through the use of inappropriate reassurance, and the excessive use of medical investigations: 'Cured yesterday of my disease, I died last night of my physician' (Matthew Prior: 1664–1721).

The standard medical training is becoming increasingly involved in high technology. Teaching of medical students has perforce to include the latest technological advances, but might also benefit from teaching students something concerning the psychology of doubt, and how illness doubt can be instilled. The method used by the authors involves encouraging groups of medical students to talk in a seminar about the well-known phenomena of 'medical student hypochondriasis'. They soon realise how common it is to imagine they have some aspect of the diseases they are studying, and can learn in this way the importance of attentional factors in symptom maintenance. Of course the students' symptoms change, as they move on to study another topic, and eventually, unlike some patients, they spontaneously 'recover'. Education of medical students in this way, and teaching the *dangers* of reassurance, using the analogy of obsessive-compulsive disorder, may be useful.

There are a number of areas where behavioural/cognitive techniques may lead in future, but it is not the aim of this book to lead into far flung territories such as those described by B.F. Skinner in his novel *Walden Two*. In that novel Skinner speculates about a Utopian future where life is wonderful, as all conditioning is perfectly understood and applied. Nevertheless, back in the realms of reality, it is worth noting one interesting direction that actual psychological research is taking (Seligman, 1989): it has been found that the way a person thinks about themselves can influence the success or failure of their behaviour. 'Optimistic' thinking about oneself predicts better grades at university, higher production in workers, and higher athletic achievement in runners and swimmers. These results in exploring 'explanatory style' have been subsumed by Seligman as: 'The future mission of cognitive therapy: making the well better'.

Appendix 1

Relaxation training

Relaxation training has a long history but the method of carrying it out, and in particular the time spent on it has been drastically reduced over the years. When described by Jacobson (1938), one to nine hour-long daily sessions were advocated up to a total of 56 sessions. Wolpe (1958) advocated a training programme that could be completed in six 20-minute sessions, with two 15-minute daily home practice sessions between training sessions. The present authors advise one 20-minute session, which is tape-recorded at the time. The tape is then given to the patient for daily home practice sessions for two weeks, after which he attends to report progress and discuss any difficulties, before entering the next phase of treatment, for which the relaxation training has usually been the prelude. Tape recorded relaxation in general is often ineffective, but it is useful when tapes are specifically made for the patient, as described, and this results in much saving of therapist's time.

Indications

Originally, relaxation was a crucial part of systematic desensitisation, but as described in chapter 1, that treatment is only of historic importance now. It still has a role in the treatment of non-phobic anxiety, where a session of relaxation training followed by homework practice can give the patient a coping skill to employ. In this way it is part of the package of treatments described in chapter 11. It also has a role in the treatment of obsessional ruminations by thought-stopping (see chapter 4). Before carrying out the instruction to 'stop' the obsessional thought, it is useful if the patient is relaxed, as it is then easier for the patient to focus their mind on this task. There are many other times when relaxation forms part of the total treatment plan, for example in the management of insomnia, and other problems in behavioural medicine (chapter 13), and as part of social skills training (chapter 7).

Procedure

The procedure begins with an explanation to the patient of the value of relaxation. It worth explaining that anxiety can cause muscular contraction, and this contraction often serves to increase anxiety and may bring about symptoms. It is also worth stressing that relaxation is not a natural ability for people in our culture, but that it can be learnt just as they may have learnt other skills such as driving a car. In the same way that learning to drive a car takes time and practice, relaxation training will take time and practice to accomplish this worthwhile ability.

Next the physical setting for relaxation is established. A quiet room, a comfortable chair with armrests and headrest are the basic minimal requirements. It is useful to have a footstool for the patient to put his feet up, and it may be necessary to ask him to remove any tight fitting clothing (e.g. necktie), shoes and spectacles.

It is explained that the aim is to contract each main muscle group in turn, and then to allow that muscle group to relax. In this way the patient becomes aware of each muscle group and also aware of any particular focus of tension, which is then dissolved by relaxation. The therapist uses modelling particularly at the start of the training, for example showing the correct way to contract the biceps, and then asking the patient to do likewise. It is usual to begin with the dominant side of the body, which is the right hand side for most people. It is also worth asking about any particular tension symptoms the patient has at the start of treatment, as particular attention can then be given to those areas. After this introduction the relaxation instructions begin:

Settle back in the chair as comfortably as you can . . . we shall then start with relaxation of your arms . . . this begins with contraction of the right biceps muscle . . . hold the contraction of the biceps for a few moments now until I tell you to stop (*about 7 seconds*). Now relax the biceps by gradually straightening out your arm and resting it on the armrest of the chair . . . now focus on the feeling of relaxation in that muscle . . . try to just think of your right biceps and nothing else for the moment (*about 15 seconds*). Next I want you to contract your forearm muscles . . . do this by making a fist with your right hand and holding it until I tell you to stop (*about 7 seconds*). Now let your fingers gradually straighten out and rest your hand over the armrest of the chair . . . focus now on the feeling of relaxation in your forearm and hand (*about 15 seconds*). Now I am going to repeat these exercises in the same way for the other arm so that both arms become completely relaxed (*Repeat as above for left arm*).

Now we will carry on with relaxation of your face and neck. Begin with the scalp muscles at the top of your head . . . contract these by raising your eyebrows towards the ceiling and holding that until I ask you to stop (*about 7 seconds*). Now let your eyebrows go to the resting position and concentrate instead on the feeling of relaxation in your scalp (*about 15 seconds*). Now think of the muscles used to close your eyes and activate these by closing your eyes until I ask you to stop (*about 7 seconds*). Now let your eyelids relax so that they are kept closed by their own weight alone . . . concentrate on this feeling of relaxation (*about 15 seconds*). Next concentrate on the muscles used to close your jaws and activate these by closing your jaws tightly until I ask you to stop (*about 7 seconds*). Now let your jaw go completely slack and concentrate on that . . . check that you are not contracting your jaw by checking with your tongue that your teeth are just a few millimetres apart (*wait about 15 seconds*). Now think of the large muscles at the back of your neck . . . contract these by pushing your head into the backrest of the chair until I ask you to stop (*about 7 seconds*) . . . now let those muscles relax by just letting your head remain there under the force of gravity alone and concentrate on that (*about 15 seconds*).

Now we will relax your chest, and abdomen or 'tummy' muscles. Begin by taking in a deep breath and hold it (*about 5 seconds*) and then slowly breathe out relaxing as you do so. Now repeat this slow breathing a few times. (*Therapist observes to check the breathing rate is correct and provides feedback, and modelling to the patient as necessary*).

To contract your abdominal muscles imagine you are punching yourself in the tummy . . . this makes you pull in these muscles . . . hold that contraction until I tell you to stop (*about 5 seconds*). Now let these muscles go slack and concentrate on that feeling for a few moments (*about 15 seconds*).

Next we shall concentrate on your thighs and calves, followed by complete body relaxation. Begin by raising your right leg off the footstool with the knee straight . . . keep it about three inches above the footstool until I tell you to lower it (*about 5 seconds*) . . . now lower your leg slowly and then concentrate on the feeling of relaxation at the top of your thigh (*about 15 seconds*). Next contract your calf muscle on the right by pulling up your foot on that side so that your toes go up towards your head . . . hold that contraction for a few moments (*about 5 seconds*). Now let your foot drop back to the resting position and concentrate on the relaxation in that calf muscle (*about 15 seconds*). *The thigh and calf exercises are now repeated for the left-hand side.*

Keep relaxing your whole body now for a while. To assist in this I am going to name each of the parts we have just relaxed, but this time instead of contracting anything just think as hard as you can of the muscles involved, and make sure that you are not contracting any muscles . . . when you are ready, begin by thinking of your right biceps . . . now right forearm . . . now left biceps . . . now left forearm . . . good . . . now switch your attention to your scalp muscles . . . now check your eyelids are lightly closed . . . now check your jaw muscles . . . then focus on the large muscles at the back of your neck . . .

Next check that you are taking nice slow easy breaths . . . and your abdomen is completely relaxed. Now check the muscles at the top of your right leg . . . now the calf on the right hand side. Now do the same with the other leg starting with the thigh . . . and then the calf on the left side. Your whole body should now be completely relaxed. Just enjoy the feeling of relaxation in those muscles as you become more deeply and completely relaxed.

The patient is told the training exercise is over, and instructed to remain relaxed for a further five minutes. Any questions about the procedure should now be dealt with. Patients often say they feel sleepy, and should be advised that it is not the aim of relaxation therapy to induce sleep, and this should be guarded against, unless of course it is for treatment of insomnia. They often confuse relaxation with hypnosis, and should be told that hypnosis is not the method used. The therapist should guard against the over use of suggestion during relaxation in order to obviate this problem. Some patients show the paradoxical effect of *increased* anxiety during relaxation. This may be due to the procedure allowing attention to focus on internal cues for anxiety. An explanation can be given along these lines, but may show the procedure is contraindicated in those few patients.

The patient is now given the tape recording that was made during the session, and asked to play it daily at home for two weeks before attending for the next appointment.

Appendix 2

Rating Scales

A2.1 Fear Questionnaire

Name .... Age .... Sex .... Date ....

Pre./Post./1m/
3m/6m

Choose a number from the scale below to show how much you would
avoid each of the situations listed below because of fear or other
unpleasant feelings. Then write the number you choose in the box
opposite each situation.

0——1——2——3——4——5——6——7——8
| would not | slightly | definitely | markedly | always |
| avoid it | avoid it | avoid it | avoid it | avoid it |

1. Main phobia you want treated (describe in you own words) –
   .... ☐
2. Injections or minor surgery .... ☐
3. Eating or drinking with other people .... ☐
4. Hospitals .... ☐
5. Travelling alone by bus or coach .... ☐
6. Walking alone in busy streets .... ☐
7. Being watched or stared at .... ☐
8. Going into crowded shops .... ☐
9. Talking to people in authority .... ☐
10. Sight of blood .... ☐
11. Being criticized .... ☐
12. Going alone far from home .... ☐
13. Thought of injury or illness .... ☐
14. Speaking or acting to an audience .... ☐
15. Large open spaces .... ☐
16. Going to the dentist .... ☐
17. Other situations (describe) .... ☐

☐ ☐ ☐ ☐
Ag + B1 + Soc = Total
2–16

Now choose a number from the scale below to show how much you are
troubled by each problem listed, and write the number in the box opposite.

0——1——2——3——4——5——6——7——8
| hardly | slightly | definitely | markedly | very severely |
| at all | troublesome | troublesome | troublesome | troublesome |

18. Feeling miserable or depressed .... ☐
19. Feeling irritable or angry .... ☐
20. Constant tension wherever I happen to be .... ☐
21. Sudden surges of panic regardless of where I am .... ☐
22. Upsetting thoughts coming into your mind .... ☐
23. Other feelings (describe) .... ☐

Total ☐

How would you rate the present state of your main problem on the scale below?

0——2——3——4——5——6——7——8
phobias	slightly	definitely	markedly	very severely
absent	disturbing/	disturbing/	disturbing/	disturbing/
	not really	disabling	disabling	disabling
	disabling			

Please circle one number between 0 and 8

Reprinted, with permission, from *Behavioural Psychotherapy* by I. M. Marks (1986) and
also from *Behaviour Research and Therapy* by I. M. Marks & A. M. Mathews (1979)

* A2.2 Compulsion Checklist

Name .... Hosp. No. ..... Date .... 19 ...

INSTRUCTIONS: The following are a list of activities which people with your kind of problem sometimes have difficulty with. Please answer each question by putting a tick under the appropriate number

0 – 'I have no problems with activity—takes me about the same time as an average person. I do not need to repeat it or avoid it.'

1 – 'This activity takes me about twice as long as most people, or I have to repeat it twice or tend to avoid it.'

2 – 'This activity takes me about three times as long as most people, or I have to repeat it three or more times, or I usually avoid it.'

3 – 'I am unable to complete or attempt activity.'

0	1	2	3	ACTIVITY
				Having a bath or shower
				Washing hands and face
				Care of hair (e.g. washing, combing, brushing)
				Brushing teeth
				Dressing and undressing
				Using toilet to urinate
				Using toilet to defaecate
				Touching people or being touched
				Handling waste or waste bins
				Washing clothes
				Washing dishes
				Handling or cooking food
				Cleaning the house
				Keeping things tidy
				Bed making
				Cleaning shoes
				Touching door handles
				Touching your genitals, petting or sexual intercourse
				Visiting a hospital
				Switching lights and taps on or off
				Locking or closing doors or windows
				Using electrical appliances (e.g. heaters)
				Doing arithmetic or accounts
				Getting to work
				Doing your work
				Writing
				Form filling
				Posting letters
				Reading
				Walking down the street
				Travelling by bus, train or car
				Looking after children
				Eating in restaurants
				Going to public toilets
				Keeping appointments
				Throwing things away
				Buying things in shops
TOTAL				
				Other (fill in)

Reprinted, with permission, from *Behavioural Psychotherapy* by I. M. Marks (1986).

† **A2.3 Social Situations Questionnaire**

Name .... Hosp. No. ..... Date ...... 19 ...
This questionnaire concerns how you get on in social situations (being
with other people, talking to them, etc.).
Please rate the discomfort you experience in the situations listed, using
the following scale:

0	1	2	3	4
no discomfort	*slight discomfort*	*moderate discomfort*	*great discomfort*	*I avoid this situation*

1. Walking down the street ......
2. Going into shops ....
3. Going on public transport .....
4. Going into pubs ....
5. Going to parties ....
6. Mixing with people at work ....
7. Making friends of your own age.
8. Going out with someone of the opposite sex ....
9. Being with a group of the same sex and roughly the same age as you
10. Being with a group of both men and women the same age as you
11. Being with a group of the opposite sex the same age as you ...
12. Entertaining people in your home, lodgings, etc. ....
13. Going into restaurants or cafes
14. Going to dances, dance halls or discotheques ....
15. Being with older people ......
16. Being with younger people ....
17. Going into a room full of people

18. Meeting strangers ....
19. Being with people you don't know very well ....
20. Being with friends
21. Making the first move in starting up a friendship ....
22. Making ordinary decisions affecting others (e.g. what to do together in the evening)
23. Being with only one other
24. Getting to know people in depth
25. Taking the initiative in keeping a conversation going ....
26. Looking at people directly in the eyes ....
27. Disagreeing with what other people are saying and putting forward your own views ......
28. People standing or sitting very close to you ....
29. Talking about yourself and your feelings in conversation ....
30. People looking at you ....

Reprinted, with permission, from *Behavioural Psychotherapy* by I. M. Marks (1986).

References

Abramson, L. Y., Seligman, M. E. P. & Teasdale, J. (1978). Learned helplessness in humans: critique and reformulation. *Journal of Abnormal Psychology*, **87**, 32–48.

American Psychiatric Association (1987). *Diagnostic and Statistical Manual of Mental Disorders*. edn., revised. Washington DC: American Psychiatric Association.

Argyle, M. & Kendon, A. (1967). The experimental analysis of social performance. In *Advances in Experimental Social Psychology*, vol. 3, ed. L. Berkowitz, pp. New York: Academic Press.

Arrindell, W. A. & Emmelkamp, P. M. G. (1986). Marital adjustment, intimacy and needs in female agoraphobics and their partners. *British Journal of Psychiatry*, **149**, 592–602.

Ayllon, T. & Azrin, N. (1968). *The Token Economy*. New York: Appleton Century Crofts.

Azrin, N. H., Naster, B. J. & Jones, R. (1973). Reciprocity counselling: a rapid learning based procedure for marital counselling. *Behaviour Research and Therapy*, **11**, 365–82.

Azrin, N. H. & Nunn, R. G. (1973). Habit reversal: A method of eliminating nervous habits and tics. *Behaviour Research and Therapy*, **11**, 619–28.

Balint, M. (1957). *The Doctor, His Patient and the Illness*. London: Pitman Medical

Bancroft, J. (1983). *Human Sexuality and its Problems*. Edinburgh: Churchill Livingstone.

Bandura, A. (1971). *Principles of Behaviour Modification*. London: Holt, Rinehart & Winston.

Barsky, A. J. (1989). *Cognitive-educational Approaches to Hypochondriasis*. Paper to World Congress of Cognitive Therapy: Oxford.

Beck, A. T., Rial, W. Y. & Rickels, K. (1974). Short form of depression inventory: cross validation. *Psychological Reports*, **34**, 1184–6.

Beck, A. T. (1978). *Depression Inventory*. Philadelphia: Center for Cognitive Therapy.

Beck, A. T. & Emery, G. (1985). *Anxiety Disorders and Phobias: A Cognitive Perspective*. New York: Basic Books.

Beck, A. T., Rush, J. A., Shaw, B. F. & Emery, G. (1979). *Cognitive Therapy of Depression*. New York: The Guilford Press.

Bellack, A. S. & Herson, M. (1979). *Research and Practice in Social Skills Training*. New York: Plenum.

Benkelfat, C., Murphy, D. L., Zohar, J., Hill, J.L., Grover, G. & Insel, T. R. (1989). Clomipramine in obsessive-compulsive disorder. *Archives of General Psychiatry*, **46**, 23–8.

Bennett, D. H. (1978). Social forms of psychiatric treatment, In *Schizophrenia: Towards a New Synthesis*. ed. J. K. Wing London: Academic Press.

Bernstein, D. A. & Borkovec, T. D. (1973). *Progressive Relaxation Training: A Manual for the Helping Professions*. Champaign Ill: Research Press.

Blackburn, I. M. (1987). *Coping with Depression*. Edinburgh: Chambers.

Blackburn, I. M., Funson, K. M. & Bishop, S. (1986). A two year naturalistic follow-up of depressed patients treated with cognitive therapy, pharmacotherapy and a combination of both. *Journal of Affective Disorders*, **10**, 67–75.

Borkovec, T. D. (1982). Insomnia. *Journal of Consulting and Clinical Psychology*, **50**, 880–95.

British National Formulary (1990). London: British Medical Association.

Brown, G. W. & Harris, T. (1978). *Social Origins of Depression*. London: Tavistock.

Butler, G., Cullington, A., Hibbert, G., Klimes, I. & Gelder, M. (1987). Anxiety management for persistent generalised anxiety. *British Journal of Psychiatry*, **151**, 535–42.

Clark, D. M. (1988). A cognitive model of panic attacks. In *Panic: Psychological Perspectives*, ed. S. J. Rachman & J. Maser, Hillsdale, NJ: Erlbaum.

Clark, D. M., Salkovskis, P. M. & Chalkley, A. J. (1985). Respiratory control as a treatment for panic attacks. *Journal of Behavior Therapy and Experimental Psychiatry*, **16**, 23–30.

Crowe, M. J. (1978). Conjoint marital therapy: a controlled outcome study. *Psychological Medicine*, **8**, 623–36.

Crowe, M. J., Gillan, P., & Golombok, S. (1981). Form and content in the conjoint treatment of sexual dysfunction: a controlled study. *Behaviour Research and Therapy*, **19**, 47–54.

Delvin, D. (1974). *The Book of Love*. London: New English Library.

Elkin, I., Shea, T., Watkins, J. T., Imber, S. D., *et al.* (1989) National Institute of Mental Health treatment of depression collaborative research program. *Archives of General Psychiatry*, **46**, 971–82.

Ellis, A. (1962) *Reason and Emotion in Pschotherapy*. New York: Lyle Stuart.

Ellis, A. & Harper, R. A. (1975) *A New Guide to Rational Living*. Englewood Cliffs, NJ: Prentice-Hall.

Emmelkamp, P. M. G. & Wessels, H. (1975). Flooding in imagination v flooding *in vivo* in agoraphobics. *Behaviour Research and Therapy*, **13**, 7–15.

Falloon, I. R. H. (1985). *Family Management of Schizophrenia*. Baltimore: The Johns Hopkins University Press.

Falloon, I. R. H., Boyd, J. L. & McGill, C. W. (1984). *Family Care of Schizophrenia*. New York: Guilford.

Feldman, R. G. & Norman, L. P. (1976). Identity of emotional triggers in epilepsy. *Journal of Nervous and Mental Disease*, **162**, 345–53.

Freud, S. (1917). *Mourning and Melancholia*. In Standard Edition, *Collected Works*, Vol. 14. London: Hogarth.

Freud, S. (1955). *Studies on Hysteria*. In the Standard Edition of the *Complete Psychological Works*, Vol. 2. London: Hogarth.

Friedman, D. (1968). The treatment of impotence by brietal relaxation therapy. *Behaviour Research and Therapy*, **6**, 257–61.

Garner, A. (1980). *Conversationally Speaking*. McGraw-Hill: New York.

Gauthier, J. & Marshall, W. L. (1977). Grief: A cognitive-behavioural analysis. *Cognitive Therapy and Research*, **1**, 39–44.

Gelder, M. G., Marks, I. M. & Wolff, H. H. (1967). Desensitization and psychotherapy in the treatment of phobic states: a controlled enquiry. *British Journal of Psychiatry*, **113**, 53–73.

Ghosh, A. (1981). *Therapeutic Interaction and Outcome in Phobia (Doctoral Dissertation)*. London: Institute of Psychiatry.

Ghosh, A., Marks, I. M. & Carr, A. C. (1988). Therapist contact and outcome of self-exposure treatment for phobias: a controlled study. *British Journal of Psychiatry*, **152**, 234–8.

Gray, J. A. (1987). Interaction between drugs and behaviour therapy. In *Theoretical Foundations of Behaviour Threrapy*, ed. H. J. Eysenck & I. Martin, New York: Plenum.

Hafner, R. J. (1977). The husbands of agoraphobic women and their influence on treatment and outcome. *British Journal of Psychiatry*, **131**, 289–94.

Hafner, R. J. & Marks, I. M. (1976). Exposure *in vivo* of agoraphobics: Contribution of diazepam, group exposure, and anxiety evocation. *Psychological Medicine*, **6**, 71–88.

Hall, J. N., Baker, R. D. & Hutchinson, K. (1977) A controlled evaluation of token economy procedures with chronic schizophrenic patients. *Behaviour Research and Therapy*, **15**, 261–83.

Hamilton, M. (1959). A rating scale for anxiety. *British Journal of Medical Psychology*, **32**, 50–5.

Hand, I., Lamontagne, Y. & Marks, I. M. (1974). Group exposure (flooding) *in vivo* for agoraphobia. *British Journal of Psychiatry*, **124**, 588–602.

Haslam, M. T. (1965). The treatment of psychogenic dyspareunia by reciprocal inhibition. *British Journal of Psychiatry*, **111**, 280–2.

Hawton, K. (1985). *Sex Therapy: A Practical Guide*. Oxford: Oxford University Press.

Hollon, S. D., Yuason, V. B., Weiner, M. J., *et al.* (1984). Combined cognitive pharmacotherapy vs. cognitive therapy alone in the treatment of depressed outpatients. Unpublished manuscript. Minneapolis, Minnesota. (cited in Paykel, E. S., 1989)

Hoogduin, C. A. L. & Hoogduin, W. A. (1983). Outpatient treatment of obsessive-compulsive disorder. *Behaviour Research and Therapy*, **22**, 455–9.

Horney, K. (1950). *Neurosis and Human Growth: The Struggle Toward Self-realisation*. New York: Norton and Co.

Jacobson, E. (1938). *Progressive Relaxation*. Chicago: University of Chicago Press.

Jacobson, N. (1981). Behavioral marital therapy. In *Handbook of Family Therapy*, ed. A. S. Gurman & D. P. Kniskern. New York: Brunner/Mazel Inc.

Jacobson, N. S. & Gurman, A. S. (1986). *Clinical Handbook of Marital Therapy*. New York: The Guilford Press.

Janet, P. (1903). *Les Obsessions et la Psychasthenie*. Paris: Baillière.

Janet, P. (1925). *Psychological Healing*. Trans. Eden and Cedar Paul. London: George Allen and Unwin.

Jenner, E. (1798). *An inquiry into the causes and effects of the variolae vaccine, a disease discovered in some of the West Counties of England, particularily Gloucestershire, and known by the name of cowpox*. Printed for the author: Sampson Low.

Johnston, D. W. (1984). Biofeedback, relaxation and related procedures in the treatment of psychophysiological disorders. In *Health care and human behaviour*, ed. A. Steptoe & A. Mathews, pp. 267–300. London: Academic Press.

Johnston, D., Lancashire, M., Mathews, A. M., Munby, M., Shaw, P. M. & Gelder, M. G. (1976). Imaginal flooding and exposure to real phobic situations: changes during treatment. *British Journal of Psychiatry*, **129**, 372–7.

Kaplan, H.S. (1976). *The Illustrated Manual of Sex Therapy*. London: Souvenir Press.

Kasvikis, Y. & Marks, I. M. (1988). Clomipramine, self-exposure, and therapist-accompanied exposure in obsessive-compulsive ritualisers: two-year follow-up. *Journal of Anxiety Disorders*, **2**, 291–8.

Klein, D. F. (1964). Delineation of two drug responsive anxiety syndromes. *Psychopharmacologia*, **5**, 397–408.

Kuhn, T. H. (1970). *The Structure of Scientific Revolutions*. Chicago: The University of Chicago Press.

Kuipers, L. (1979). Schizophrenia and the family. Part 1: The problems of relatives. In *Community Care for the Mentally Disabled*, J. K. Wing & R. Olsen, pp. Oxford: Oxford University Press.

Latimer, P. R. (1981). Irritable bowel syndrome: a behavioural model. *Behaviour Research and Therapy*, **19**, 475–83.

Lazarus, A. A. (1963). The treatment of chronic frigidity by systematic desensitisation. *Journal of Nervous and Mental Disorders*, **136**, 272–8.

Lazarus, A. A. (1973). Multimodal behaviour therapy: treating the 'Basic ID'. *Journal of Nervous and Mental Disorders*, **156**, 404–11.

Leff, J. and Vaughn, C. (1985). *Expressed Emotion in Families*. New York: The Guilford Press.

Leonard, H. L., Swedo, S., Rappoport, J. L., *et al.* (1988). Treatment of childhood obsessive-compulsive disorder with clomipramine and desmethylimipramine: a double blind crossover comparison. *Psychopharmacology Bulletin* **24**, 93–95.

Levy, R. & Meyer, V. (1971). Ritual prevention in obsessional patients. *Proceedings of the Royal Society of Medicine*, **64**, 115–20.

Lewinsohn, P. M. (1975). Behavioral study and treatment of depression. In *Progress in Behavior Modification*, vol. 1, ed. R. M. Eisler & P. M. Miller, New York: Academic Press.

Lewinsohn, P. M. & Graf, M. (1973). Pleasant activities and depression. *Journal of Consulting and Clinical Psychology*, **41**, 261–8.

Lewis, A. J. (1935). Problems of obsessional illness. *Proceedings of the Royal Society of Medicine*, **29**, 325–6.

Lieberman, S. (1978). Nineteen cases of morbid grief. *British Journal of Psychiatry*, **132**, 159–63.

Locke, J. (1693). *Some Thoughts Concerning Education*. London: Ward, Lock and Co.

Lopez-Ibor, J. J. (1966). Ensayo clinico de la monochloripramine. *Presented at the Fourth World Congress of Psychiatry*, Madrid.

Macaulay, A. J., Stern, R. S., Holmes, D. M. & Stanton, S. L. (1987). Micturition and the mind: psychological factors in the aetiology and treatment of urinary symptoms in women. *British Medical Journal*, **294**, 540–3.

Macleod, J. G. (1973) *Clinical Examination*. London: Churchill Livingstone.

McDonald, R., Sartory, G., Grey, S. J., Cobb, J., Stern, R. & Marks, I. M. (1978). Effects of self-exposure instructions on agoraphobic outpatients. *Behaviour Research and Therapy*, **17**, 83–5.

Marks,I.M. (1973). The reduction of fear: towards a unifying theory. *Journal of the Canadian Psychiatric Association*, **18**, 9–12.

Marks, I. M. (1978). *Living with Fear*. New York: McGraw-Hill.

Marks, I. M. (1981). *Cure and Care of Neurosis*. New York: Wiley.

Marks, I. M. (1986). *Behavioural Psychotherapy*. Bristol: Wright.

Marks, I. M. (1987). *Fears, Phobias and Rituals*. Oxford: Oxford University Press.

Marks, I. M., Connolly, J. & Philpott, R. (1977). *Nursing in Behavioural Psychotherapy*. London: Research Series of Royal College of Nursing.

Marks, I. M., Gray, S., Cohen, D., Hill, R., Mawson, D., Ramm, E. & Stern, R. (1983). Imipramine and brief therapist-aided exposure in agoraphobics having self-exposure homework. *Archives of General Psychiatry*, **40**, 153–62.

Marks, I. M., Hodgson, R. & Rachman, S. (1975). Treatment of chronic OCD two years after *in vivo* exposure. *British Journal of Psychiatry*, **127**, 349–64.

Marks, I. M., Lelliot, P., Basoglu, M., Noshirvani, H., Monteiro, W., Cohen, D. & Kasvikis, Y. (1988). Clomipramine, self-exposure and therapist-aided exposure for obsessive-compulsive rituals. *British Journal of Psychiatry*, **152**, 522–34.

Marks, I. M. & Mathews, A. M. (1979). Brief standard self-rating for phobic patients. *Behaviour Research and Therapy*, **17**, 263–7.

Marks, I. M. & O'Sullivan, G. (1988). Drugs and psychological treatments for agoraphobia/panic and obsessive-compulsive disorders: a review. *British Journal of Psychiatry*, **153**, 650–8.

Marks, I. M., Stern, R. S., Mawson, D., Cobb, J. & McDonald, R. (1980). Clomipramine and exposure for obsessive-compulsive rituals: 1. *British Journal of Psychiatry*, **136**, 1–25.

Marquis, J. N. (1970). Orgasmic reconditioning: changing sexual object choice through controlling masturbation fantasies. *Journal of Behavior Therapy and Experimental Psychiatry*, **1**, 263–70.

Masters, W. H. & Johnson, V. E. (1966) *Human Sexual Response*. London: Churchill

Masters, W. H. & Johnson, V. E. (1970). *Human Sexual Inadequacy*. London: Churchill.

Mathews, A. M., Gelder, M. G. & Johnston, D. W. (1981). *Programmed Practice for Agoraphobia*. London: Tavistock.

Mathews, A. M., Johnston, D. W., Lancashire, M., *et al.* (1976). Imaginal flooding v. real exposure in agoraphobics: outcome. *British Journal of Psychiatry*, **129**, 362–71.

Mavissakalian, M., Turner, S. M., Michelson, L., *et al.* (1985). Tricyclic antidepressant in obsessive-compulsive disorder: antiobsessional or antidepressant agents? *American Journal of Psychiatry*, **142**, 572–6.

Mawson, D., Marks, I. M. & Ramm, E. (1982). Clomipramine and exposure for chronic OC rituals: III. Two year follow-up. *British Journal of Psychiatry*, **140**, 11–18.

Mawson, D., Marks, I. M., Ramm, E. & Stern, R. S. (1981). Guided mourning for morbid grief: a controlled study. *British Journal of Psychiatry*, **138**, 185–93.

Meichenbaum, D. (1977). *Cognitive-Behavior Modification: An Integrative Approach*. New York: Plenum Press.

Merskey, H. (1984). Too much pain. *British Journal of Hospital Medicine*, January, 63–66.

Meyer, V. & Chesser, E. S. (1970). *Behaviour Therapy in Clinical Psychiatry*. London: Penguin.

Morgan, W. P. & Goldston, S. E. (1987). *Exercise and Mental Health*. Washington DC: Hemisphere.

Murray, R. M. & Reveley, A. (1981). The genetic contribution to the neurosis. *British Journal of Hospital Medicine*, Febrary, 185–90.

Nagy, L. M., Krystal, J. H., Woods, S. W. & Charney, D. S. (1989). Clinical and medication outcome after short term Alprazolam and behavioral group treatment in panic disorder. *Archives of General Psychiatry*, **46**, 993–9.

Newell, R. (1989). *Behavioural Interventions with the Irritable Bowel Syndrome.* Paper to The Association of Behavioural Clinician's Conference: London.

Noyes, R., Anderson, D. J., Clancy, J., *et al* (1984). Diazepam and propranolol in panic disorder and agoraphobia. *Archives of General Psychiatry*, **41**, 287–92.

O'Leary, K. D. & Wilson, G. T. (1975). *Behavior Therapy: Application and Outcome.* New Jersey: Prentice-Hall.

Oswald, I. M. (1966). *Sleep.* Penguin: London.

Oswald, I. M. (1984). Insomnia. *British Journal of Hospital Medicine*, March, 219–24.

Patel, C., Marmot, M. G. & Terry, D. J. (1981). Controlled trial of biofeedback and behavioural methods in reducing mild hypertension. *British Medical Journal*, **282**, 2005–8.

Paykel, E. S. (1989). Treatment of depression. *British Journal of Psychiatry*, **155**, 754–63.

Phillips, A. & Rakusen, J. (1978). *Our Bodies Ourselves.* London: Penguin.

Premack, D. (1959). Toward empirical behavior laws: 1. Positive reinforcement. *Psychological Review*, **66**, 219–33.

Price, L. H., Goodman, W. K., Charney, D. S., *et al.* (1987). Treatment of severe obsessive-compulsive disorder with fluvoxamine. *American Journal of Psychiatry*, **144**, 1059–61.

Rachman, S., Hodgson, R. & Marks, I. M. (1971). Treatment of chronic obsessive-compulsive neurosis. *Behaviour Research and Therapy*, **9**, 237–47.

Ramsay, R. W. (1977). Behavioural approaches to bereavement. *Behaviour Research and Therapy*, **15**, 131–5.

Raphael, B. (1977). Preventative intervention with the recently bereaved. *Archives of General Psychiatry*, **34**, 1450–54.

Salkovskis, P. M. (1985). Obsessional-compulsive problems: a cognitive-behavioural analysis. *Behaviour Research and Therapy*, **25**, 571–83.

Salkovskis, P. M. & Clark, D. M. (1990). Affective responses to hyperventilation: a test of the cognitive model of panic. *Behaviour Research and Therapy*, **28**, 51–61.

Salkovskis, P. M. & Warwick, H. M. C. (1986). Morbid preoccupations, health anxiety and reassurance: a cognitive-behavioural approach to hypochondriasis. *Behaviour Research and Therapy*, **24**, 597–602.

Salkovskis, P. M. & Warwick, H. M. C. (1988). Cognitive therapy of obsessive-compulsive disorder. In *The Theory and Practice of Cognitive therapy*, ed. C. Perris, I. M. Blackburn & H. Perris, pp. 376–95. Heidelberg: Springer-Verlag.

Seligman, M. E. P. (1975). *On Depression, Development and Death.* San Francisco: W. H. Freeman.

Seligman, M. E. P. (1989). The Future Mission of Cognitive Therapy: Making the Well Better. Keynote address to World Congress of Cognitive Therapy: Oxford.

Selmi, P. M., Klein, M. H., Greist, J. H., Sorrell, S. P. & Erdman, H. P. (1990). Computer-administered cognitive-behavioural therapy for depression. *American Journal of Psychiatry*, **147**, 51–6.

Semans, J. M. (1956). Premature ejaculation: a new approach. *Southern Medical Journal*, **49**, 353–7.

Shepherd, G. (1983). Chapter 1: Introduction. In *Developments in Social Skills Training*, ed. S. Spence & G. Shepherd, London: Academic Press.

Shepherd, G. (1984). *Institutional Care and Rehabilitation*. London: Longman.

Simons, A. D., Murphy, G. E., Levine, J. L., *et al.* (1986). Cognitive therapy and pharmacotherapy for depression. *Archives of General Psychiatry*, **43**, 43–50.

Sireling, L., Cohen, D. & Marks, I. (1988). Guided mourning for morbid grief: A controlled replication. *Behavior Therapy*, **19**, 121–32.

Skinner, B. F. (1953). *Science and Human Behavior*. New York: The Free Press.

Skynner, R. & Cleese, J. (1983). *Families and How to Survive Them*. London: Methuen.

Sobell, M. B. & Sobell, L. C. (1978). *Behavioral Treatment of Alcohol Problems*. New York: Plenum.

Stampfl, T. J. & Levis, D. G. (1967). Essentials of implosive therapy: a learning theory based psychodynamic behavior therapy. *Journal of Abnormal Psychology*, **72**, 496–503.

Stern, R. S. (1975). The medical student as behavioural psychotherapist. *British Medical Journal*, **2**, 78–81.

Stern, R. S. (1978a). *Behavioural Techniques*. London: Academic Press.

Stern, R. S. (1978b). Obsessive thoughts: The problem of therapy. *British Journal of Psychiatry*, **132**, 200–5.

Stern, R. S. & Cobb, J. P. (1978). Phenomenology of obsessive-compulsive neurosis. *British Journal of Psychiatry*, **132**, 233–9.

Stern, R. S. & Marks, I. M. (1973). Brief and prolonged flooding: a comparison in agoraphobic patients. *Archives of General Psychiatry*, **28**, 270–6.

Stern, R. S., Marks, I. M., Mawson, D. & Luscombe, D. K. (1980). Clomipramine and exposure for compulsive rituals: II. Plasma levels, side effects and outcome. *British Journal of Psychiatry*, **136**, 161–6.

Stuart, R. B. (1967). Behavioral control of overeating. *Behaviour Research and Therapy*, **1**, 357–65.

Stuart, R. B. (1969). Operant-interpersonal treatment for marital discord. *Journal of Consulting and Clinical Psychology*. **33**, 675–82.

Stuart, R. B. (1973). *Premarital Counselling Inventory*. Champaign, IL: Research Press.

Stuart, R. B. (1980). *Helping Couples Change*. New York: The Guilford Press.

Suinn, R. M. & Richardson, F. (1971). Anxiety management training: a non-specific behavior therapy program for anxiety control. *Behavior Therapy*, **2**, 498–510.

Telch, M. J., Agras, W. S., Taylor, C. B., Roth, W. T. & Gallen, C. G. (1985). Combined pharmacolgical and behavioral treatment for agoraphobia. *Behaviour Research and Therapy*, **23**, 325–34.

Turner, S. M., Jacob, R.G., Beidel, D. C., *et al.* (1985). Fluoxetine treatment of obsessive-compulsive disorder. *Journal of Clinical Pharmacology*, **5**, 207–12.

Ullrich, R., Ullrich, G., Crombach, G. & Peikert, V. (1975). Three flooding procedures for agoraphobia. In *Progress in Behaviour Therapy* ed. J. C. Brengelmann, pp. 59–67. New-York: Springer-Verlag.

Vaughn, C, E. & Leff, J. P. (1976). The influence of family and social factors on the course of psychiatric illness. *British Journal of Psychiatry*, **129**, 125–37.

Wardle, J. (1990). Behaviour therapy and benzodiazepines: allies or antagonists? *British Journal of Psychiatry*, **156**, 163–8.

Watson, J. P. & Marks, I. M. (1971). Relevant and irrelevant fear in flooding – a crossover study of phobic patients. *Behavior Therapy*, **2**, 275–93.

Weissman, M. M. & Paykel, E. S. (1974). *The Depressed Woman*. Chicago: The Chicago Press.

Wing, J. K. & Morris. B. (1981). Clinical basis of rehabilitation. In *Handbook of Psychiatric Practice*, ed. J. K. Wing & B. Morris, Oxford: Oxford University Press.

Wolpe, J. & Lazarus, A. A. (1966). *Behaviour Therapy Techniques: A Guide to the Treatment of Neurosis*. Oxford: Pergamon Press.

Wolpe, J. (1958). *Psychotherapy by Reciprocal Inhibition*. Stanford: Stanford University Press.

Zilbergeld, B. (1980). *Men and Sex*. London: Fontana.

Zitrin, C. M., Klein, D. F. & Woerner, M. G. (1980). Treatment of agoraphobia with group exposure *in vivo* and imipramine. *Archives of General Psychiatry*, **37**, 63–72.

Index